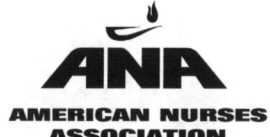

AMERICAN NURSES
ASSOCIATION

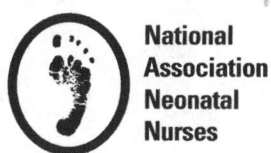

National
Association of
Neonatal
Nurses

Scope AND
Standards
OF PRACTICE

Neonatal Nursing

2ND EDITION

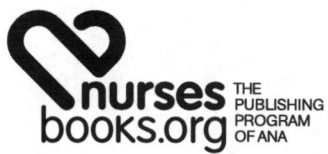

American Nurses Association
Silver Spring, Maryland
2013

Library of Congress Cataloging-in-Publication data

Neonatal nursing: scope and standards of practice/National Association of Neonatal Nurses, American Nurses Association. —2nd ed.
    p. ; cm.
Includes bibliographical references and index.
ISBN 978-1-55810-470-9 (soft cover: alk. paper)—ISBN 978-1-55810-471-6 (ebook (PDF format))—ISBN 978-1-55810-472-3 (ebook (EPUB format))—ISBN 978-1-55810-473-0 (ebook (Mobipocket format))
I. National Association of Neonatal Nurses. II. American Nurses Association.
[DNLM: 1. Neonatal Nursing—standards. WY 157.3]

618.92'00231—dc23   2012040425

The American Nurses Association (ANA) and the National Association of Neonatal Nurses (NANN) are national professional associations. This joint ANA–NANN publication (*Neonatal Nursing: Scope and Standards of Practice, Second Edition*) reflects the thinking of the practice specialty of neonatal nursing on various issues and should be reviewed in conjunction with state board of nursing policies and practices. State law, rules, and regulations govern the practice of nursing, while *Neonatal Nursing: Scope and Standards of Practice, Second Edition* guides neonatal nurses in the application of their professional skills and responsibilities.

American Nurses Association
8515 Georgia Avenue, Suite 400
Silver Spring, MD 20910-3492
1-800-274-4ANA
http://www.NursingWorld.org

Published by Nursesbooks.org
The Publishing Program of ANA
http://www.Nursesbooks.org/

ISBN-13: 978-1-55810-470-9   SAN: 851-3481   02/2013

First printing: February 2013

Contents

Acknowledgments

This document was developed by the National Association of Neonatal Nurses Scope and Standards Task Force. The task force members gratefully acknowledge the work of the previous task forces that initiated the original documents on neonatal nursing practice. The early versions of the manuscript for this edition were modified on the basis of thoughtful comments and editing suggestions made by volunteer reviewers and by the NANN Board of Directors.

This edition is dedicated to the past, present, and future families and staff of the NICU, working in partnership to benefit all babies in our care.

Contributors

National Association of Neonatal Nurses (NANN) Scope and Standards Task Force

Karen M. Kopischke, MS, RNC, NNP-BC—Chair

Annette Carley, MS, RN, NNP-BC, PNP

Kim Maryniak, MSN, BN, RNC

Linda Merritt, MSN, RNC

Susan Stang, MSN, RNC, APN

NANN Staff Liaisons

Barbara Hofmaier, MAT

Catherine Underwood, MBA, CAE

NANN Board of Directors, 2011–2012

Susan Reinarz, MSN, RN, NNP-BC—President

Cheryl Ann Carlson, PhD, APRN, NNP-BC—President-Elect

Gladys Mabey, MN, RN—Secretary-Treasurer

Lori Armstrong, MSN, RN—Immediate Past President

Julianne Dahl, MSN, RNC-NIC—Staff Nurse Director at Large

Elizabeth Damato, PhD, RNC, CPNP—Special Interest Groups Director at Large

Regina Grazel, MSN, RN, BC, APN-C—Director at Large

Debra A. Sansoucie, EdD, APRN, NNP-BC—National Association of Neonatal Nurse Practitioners (NANNP) Council Chair

Moni Snell, MSN, NNP-BC—Director at Large

Carol Wallman, MSN, RN, NNP-BC—Director at Large

American Nurses Association (ANA) Staff

Carol Bickford, PhD, RN-BC, CPHIMS—Content editor
Maureen E. Cones, Esq.—Legal counsel
Yvonne Daley Humes, MSA—Project coordinator
Eric Wurzbacher, BA—Project editor

About the American Nurses Association

The American Nurses Association (ANA) is the only full-service professional organization representing the interests of the nation's 3.1 million registered nurses through its constituent/state nurses associations and its organizational affiliates. The ANA advances the nursing profession by fostering high standards of nursing practice, promoting the rights of nurses in the workplace, projecting a positive and realistic view of nursing, and lobbying the Congress and regulatory agencies on health care issues affecting nurses and the public.

About the National Association of Neonatal Nurses

The National Association of Neonatal Nurses (NANN) supports the professional needs of neonatal nurses throughout their careers and shapes the field of neonatal nursing through excellence in practice, education, research, and professional development. The longest established professional organization for neonatal nurses, NANN provides its members a connection to the strongest and most vibrant community of neonatal nurses in the United States.

About Nursesbooks.org, The Publishing Program of ANA

Nursesbooks.org publishes books on ANA core issues and programs, including ethics, leadership, quality, specialty practice, advanced practice, and the profession's enduring legacy. Best known for the foundational documents of the profession on nursing ethics, scope and standards of practice, and social policy, Nursesbooks.org is the publisher for the professional, career-oriented nurse, reaching and serving nurse educators, administrators, managers, and researchers as well as staff nurses in the course of their professional development.

Scope of Neonatal Nursing Practice

Definition and Overview of Professional Neonatal Nursing

Neonatal nursing is the specialized practice of care for the neonate, infant, and family from birth and initial hospitalization through discharge and early follow-up care. This highly specialized nursing practice includes care of infants born prematurely and those born at term or beyond who are experiencing illness or complications following their birth, as well as newborns who remain at risk for disorders of transition and later onset of symptoms of pathology.

Medical and technological breakthroughs have expanded the ability to save extremely small and immature infants as well as profoundly ill infants, which has inevitably and extensively changed practice. With these innovations and practice changes, the nursing care needs of this population have grown. As a result, the population served has expanded to include infants during the first 2 years of life who have healthcare needs related to their neonatal period (National Association of Neonatal Nurses [NANN], 2009b).

The population served by neonatal registered nurses is diverse and increasing. According to the Centers for Disease Control and Prevention (CDC), 1 in 8 infants is born preterm, and 7% are born with low birth weight in the United States (CDC, 2006). The U.S. Department of Health and Human Services reported that in 2006, 4% of all births required assisted ventilation immediately after birth, and of those, 20% required assisted ventilation for more than 6 hours after delivery. This same report, derived from data from the 19 states that had implemented the 2003 U.S. Standard Certificate of Live Birth, reported that 6% of all infants reported were admitted to a neonatal intensive care unit (NICU) (Osterman, Martin, & Menacker, 2009). Overall infant mortality in 2012 was 6.61 infant deaths per 1,000 live births, and the leading cause of death was congenital malformations, which accounted for 20% of all deaths. The second leading cause of death was disorders related to short gestation and low birth weight, which accounted for an additional 17% of all infant deaths (Mathews & MacDorman, 2008). Data from 2005 suggested that the annual societal economic costs (medical and educational expenses and costs of lost productivity) associated with preterm birth in the United States were at least $26.2 billion (March of Dimes, 2010).

Neonatal care in the developed world tends to focus on highly technological solutions to infant mortality. In the developing world, infant mortality is an enormous problem. In some areas, more than 100 of every 1,000 live births die before the age of one (World Health Organization, 2012). The direct causes of death and disability vary considerably throughout the world, as do the causes of low birth weight and prematurity. Infant and child mortality are rising in some resource-poor areas of the world, where the challenge is to have a skilled attendant provide seamless care throughout the entire pregnancy and neonatal period, addressing the health issues prevalent in that region (WHO, 2005). The neonatal nurse practicing in these areas faces the challenge of providing lifesaving care with limited resources in the context of difficult social and governmental structures.

The numbers of critically ill infants surviving to discharge has increased, and the specialty has evolved to encompass the care of convalescing or fragile infants up to 1 year of age. The neonatal registered nurse recognizes and respects each infant as a unique, individual human being, with the right to a pain-free, developmentally supportive care environment. The nurse assists the family's adaptation to a new, highly technical environment, while encouraging attachment to and bonding with the newborn. The neonatal registered nurse recognizes the family's attachment to the newborn as crucial for the infant's physical, psychological, and emotional well-being. The neonatal registered nurse strives to empower the family through education, practice, and competence in caring for the newborn. This is achieved through promoting family-focused care, assisting parents with adapting to and gaining meaning from the neonatal experience, and fostering their independence in assuming care of the neonate/infant. This process begins at the time of birth, when the parents are taught developmentally and physiologically appropriate handling.

As the infant's physiologic status improves and the infant matures, the family is encouraged to participate in the infant's care increasingly until the time comes when the family is able to care more completely for the child.

This document is intended to identify some of the issues and trends that have an impact on the practice of professional neonatal nursing. It is not intended to restrict role development and nursing practice, but rather to frame and clarify the scope and foundation of the work of professional nurses at all levels of practice. It is intended to be used in conjunction with *Code of Ethics for Nurses with Interpretive Statements* (American Nurses Association [ANA], 2001), *Nursing's Social Policy Statement: The Essence of the Profession* (ANA, 2010b), and *Nursing: Scope and Standards of Practice, Second Edition* (ANA, 2010a).

The scope of neonatal nursing practice describes the "who," "what," "where," "why," "when," and "how" of nursing practice within this specialty area. These descriptors create a complete picture of the dynamic and complex practice of neonatal nursing. The total scope of neonatal nursing practice that an individual nurse engages in is influenced by education, experience, role, and population served (ANA, 2010a).

History of Neonatal Nursing

The roots of neonatal nursing are in the care of mothers and babies throughout history. Midwives and experienced female elders have cared for women through pregnancy and delivery and shortly after delivery for centuries. However, the focus of their care was clearly on the woman, and infant mortality was very high. Modern neonatal nursing as a subspecialty began with the invention of the incubator in 1878 by the French obstetrician Étienne Tarnier. In 1884, Tarnier also invented a small tube for the administration of gavage feedings (Raju, 2011). These two interventions revolutionized the care of sick and preterm infants. Two decades later, "premature baby shows" began in Europe and the United States. These shows were quite successful and eventually led to the establishment of a Premature Infant Station at Michael Reese Medical Center in Chicago in 1914. This unit was run by Julian Hess, a pediatrician, and Evelyn Lundeen, the head nurse. They achieved unparalleled survival rates, in part because of rigorous attention to the details of environmental control, asepsis, and feeding (Raju, 2011). These facets of care—thermoregulation, infection control, and nutrition—underpin the care we provide today.

As the 20th century unfolded, the options available for care of newborns expanded. Blood transfusions, intravenous fluids, and ventilators all became commonplace. In 1950, the first federal grant funding the Premature Institute program was allocated to train hospitals in caring for this group of infants. Despite this, in 1963, President John Kennedy's newborn son, who was born at 4 lbs 10 oz and 34 weeks' gestation, died of respiratory distress syndrome. He was 39 hours old ("The presidency," 1963). This family tragedy was widely reported and illustrated to the public that tremendous work in the field remained to be done.

In the ensuing years, basic research into the physiology of the premature infant has led to an explosion of drugs, devices, and treatments for even the tiniest and most immature of infants. As these treatment options became prevalent and survival of smaller and sicker infants became common, neonatal nurses developed innovative methods of improving infant outcomes. Developmental care and skin-to-skin care have become essential components of the nursing care provided to these infants. Nurses have been instrumental in developing methods to assess and treat pain in the infant. The modern NICU employs evidence-based nursing and medical care in a collaborative manner.

Underlying Assumptions of Neonatal Nursing

The following assumptions were made in the development of *Neonatal Nursing: Scope and Standards of Practice*:

- The standards focus primarily on the process of providing nursing care to newborns/infants and their families.

- The healthcare facility has the responsibility to provide a sufficient number of qualified registered nurses to deliver safe and effective neonatal nursing care.

- Nursing care is individualized to meet the unique needs of each newborn/infant and family.

- The nurse considers and respects the family's goals and preferences when developing and implementing a plan of care.

- The nurse respects culture and diversity in all aspects of newborn/infant and family care and administers nursing care accordingly.

- The nurse respects the privacy rights of the newborn/infant and family and manages all information accordingly.

- The nurse provides information to the family so informed decisions can be made regarding the care of the newborn/infant and family.

- The nurse functions within the Nurse Practice Act of the state and the established policies and procedures as described by the healthcare institution in which the nurse is practicing.

- The nurse works in coordination and collaboration with other healthcare providers to render care to the newborn/infant and family.

- The nurse strives to provide the highest quality of care while utilizing available resources.

- The nurse strives to promote optimal outcomes within the confines of current practice standards.

- The nurse strives to ensure use of evidence-based care when possible and advocates for research in areas lacking evidence to support practice.

- The family is the integral unit for care.

Practice Characteristics of Neonatal Nursing

The unique physiology of the neonate and the care of her or his family is the foundation upon which neonatal nursing is based. Neonatal registered nurses understand the complex conditions and disease processes affecting a patient population that includes those born at a range of gestational ages. The transition to extra-uterine life is a unique period of rapid physiologic change, found only in this age group. Critically ill neonates may include those born prematurely with incompletely developed or functional organ systems, those suffering the effects of impaired transition to postnatal life, and infants with a variety of congenital abnormalities. The newborn infant's ability to accomplish the complicated task of transition to extra-uterine life is influenced by gestation, presence of physical defects, perinatal risks such as chronic maternal illness or drug exposure, infection, and other factors. Infants who have required intensive neonatal support for early illness or prematurity are at additional risk for long-term complications such as chronic lung disease, impaired growth, and poor neurodevelopmental outcomes. The interplay between the infant's relative immaturity, genetic background, and the complications associated with lifesaving treatment modalities can produce physiologic changes that are unique to this population.

Maternal health and disease can have profound effects on the developing fetus. Placental function influences growth and development both in utero and ex utero. Placental dysfunction can produce a myriad of effects in the infant, which can in turn produce significant complications, both short-term and long-term. A growing body of evidence shows that adult diseases can have their origins in fetal pathology (Devaskar & Calkins, 2011). Neonatal nurses are aware of the potential effects of maternal health on the developing human and evaluate the infant for subtle signs of these complications in an attempt to ameliorate these problems.

The challenges to nursing care that these maternal and neonatal factors present require a skill set that is highly specialized and an extremely high level of vigilance and attention to minute detail. In caring for newborn infants, the neonatal registered nurse recognizes the importance of holistic care and supports the family's adaptive coping skills in this setting.

The care of infants in the NICU must be provided in a manner that is age appropriate. Age-appropriate care for infants includes attention to five core measures: protected sleep, pain and stress assessment, age-appropriate activities of daily living, family-focused care, and the healing environment (Coughlin, 2011). These core measures and other specific tenets that form the framework for neonatal nursing practice include the following.

Continuous Assessment

Vigilance—reflected in continuous assessment and monitoring of the fragile, preverbal infant—is vital. The neonatal registered nurse detects subtle changes in the infant's physiologic status and communicates these changes to the appropriate interprofessional team members, including physicians; advanced practice registered nurses; case managers; laboratory technicians; occupational, physical, and respiratory therapists; nutritionists; social workers; and child-life specialists. The critical care skills of continuous assessment and response to findings are employed in the first moments of life and then throughout the infant's convalescence. For instance, early identification of the subtle symptoms of hypothermia or of increased apnea, bradycardia, and lethargy in a previously stable infant can lead to the early identification of sepsis in this population.

The goal is to provide safe, timely, and comprehensive intervention and care for the fragile newborn and family, within the context of larger systems and environments. The neonatal registered nurse identifies and treats pain and prevents suffering through management of the infant's discomfort, employing a variety of both pharmacologic and nonpharmacologic interventions (Walden & Gibbins, 2008).

Developmental Care

The neonatal registered nurse provides care for medically fragile infants who may be physiologically and developmentally immature. Infants in neonatal care units face the dual challenge of meeting appropriate developmental milestones and enduring a period of critical illness. The neonatal registered nurse provides a therapeutic environment that utilizes evidence-based practices favoring optimal developmental outcomes and supporting physiologic stability. Ultimately, the goal is to maximize outcomes while supporting the infant's development, thereby enhancing the infant's growth and neurodevelopmental potential. The neonatal registered nurse utilizes knowledge of the dynamic relationship between innate behaviors and the environment to shape the care that is provided, allowing for wake-sleep cycles, circadian rhythms, and appropriate sensory experiences, and fostering homeostasis (Gardner & Goldson, 2011). Sleep plays a critical role in the development of synapses, in learning, and in memory. The protection of sleep is fundamental to the care provided (Coughlin, 2011).

Health Promotion

In planning and providing care, the neonatal registered nurse considers all aspects of the infant's health, including preventive health care, growth, and anticipatory guidance. The neonatal registered nurse closely assesses the infant's physiologic status, develops a specialized plan of care, and evaluates the infant's response. The neonatal registered nurse devises, coordinates, and executes an individualized plan of care for the newborn, both during the period of acute illness and during convalescence, revising plans as needed and continually evaluating responses from the infant and the family (Ikuta & Beauman, 2011). Activities of daily living are provided in an age-appropriate manner so that positioning, handling, feeding, and routine care affect the infant's physiologic status positively (Coughlin, 2011).

Environment

The neonatal registered nurse recognizes the significant effects of the environment on the health of the newborn. These effects, such as challenges with thermoregulation, can be seen within the first "golden hour" of life, but also are seen throughout the infant's hospitalization as the infant's clinical condition and environmental requirements change. The nurse strives to eliminate or minimize negative iatrogenic effects for the infant and to provide a nurturing environment. This may include, but is not limited to, providing uninterrupted sleep periods, maintaining a neutral thermal environment, providing comfort and reducing stress, controlling the ambient lighting and noise level in the unit, and minimizing the risk of infection (Kenner & McGrath, 2010). The neonatal registered nurse promotes positive family–infant interaction by providing opportunities for touch, holding, and skin-to-skin care, optimizing breast or bottle feeding, and encouraging active participation in the infant's daily care needs.

Family-Centered Care

Neonatal registered nurses recognize the family as an integral part of effective care delivery, and they honor the partnership between families and the neonatal team. Care practices consider dignity and respect for family beliefs and culture, along with the need for accurate, complete, and timely information sharing. The neonatal registered nurse encourages parental presence and direct involvement in caregiving to maximize physiologic stability and developmental outcomes and prepare for discharge. Throughout the infant's hospitalization, the family members are encouraged to increase their participation in hands-on care as appropriate to the infant's physiologic status. The neonatal registered nurse recognizes that this evolution in parental care improves the ability of the family to confidently care for the infant as he or she transitions to home. Families are encouraged to collaborate in both individualized care of the newborn and programmatic development benefiting all neonates (Griffin, 2006).

On occasion, newborns experience life-limiting conditions. Neonatal registered nurses play an essential role in helping the infant and her or his family receive dignified, individualized, culturally sensitive care. The neonatal registered nurse is sensitive to optimizing opportunities for infant–family experiences in the time remaining, including but not limited to holding the infant, introducing the infant to the extended family, or taking the infant home with perinatal hospice support (NANN, 2010b).

Culturally Sensitive Care

Cultural competence is the process of delivering health care within the context of a patient family's values, beliefs, and customs (Barksdale, 2009). The neonatal registered nurse provides culturally sensitive care to the infant and family by acknowledging the family's unique cultural needs while caring for that infant. Culturally competent care in an increasingly diverse and multicultural society is an ongoing developmental process. Understanding the family's core cultural dynamics, the meaning of the illness, and the social context in which this is all occurring assists the neonatal registered nurse in delivering the care the infant requires (Siegel, Gardner, & Dickey, 2011). Family-focused, culturally appropriate care can eliminate potential barriers to health care for the family and is essential for the infant's well-being. Whenever feasible, the cultural practices and beliefs of the infant's family are respected and accommodated by the neonatal registered nurse and the multidisciplinary team. Examples include assisting the family to arrange for the baptism of their infant, bathing, and unique rituals (Kenner & Sudia-Robinson, 2007).

Spiritual Care

The neonatal registered nurse plays an integral role in helping families cope with the conflicting emotions experienced in the NICU. The nurse recognizes and helps families acknowledge, address, and cope with the variety of emotions that coexist, including hope and joy, grief and loss, anger and disappointment, and helplessness and isolation. Hospitalization of the sick newborn is recognized as family crisis, involving all members of the family. Protracted neonatal illness will extend the period of family stress. The neonatal registered nurse understands that grieving is an individual process and occurs in stages. The neonatal registered nurse recognizes and respects religious and spiritual family practices, while conveying acceptance, openness, and availability. Spiritual support is necessary regardless of the infant's outcome. The neonatal registered nurse assists the family and the infant at the end of life in whatever ways possible (NANN, 2010b). In some instances, families may experience complicated situations in which decisions about the care of their infant are necessary. The decisions may be difficult for them to make or difficult for care providers to understand. Parents and care providers who are involved in these situations may benefit from supportive care (Kavanaugh & Wheeler, 2007).

Ethical Decision-Making

In practice, the neonatal registered nurse is often challenged with ethical issues. Technological advances have moved us in 50 years from "nothing can be done" to "everything must be done" to "parents can choose" to "are we overdoing?" (Catlin, 2009). Ethical dilemmas exist because disparate individuals propose different courses of action that may result in quite different outcomes. Ethical issues may arise from past actions or proposed actions. Where ethical issues exist, the solution may result in moral distress for the care providers involved. The individual nurse who is involved in these scenarios must avoid a paternalistic attitude in her or his relationship with the family and infant (Williams & Sudia-Robinson, 2007).

Strategies for resolution of conflict and ethical issues are important skills for nurses in the NICU. It is clear that one of the key skills for the resolution of an ethical issue is communication. The neonatal registered nurse works to develop this skill throughout her or his career. In addition, the nurse identifies any precipitating factors that produce or exacerbate the ethical issue. Following identification of the problem, the nurse analyzes the problem; this analysis may include the participation of interdisciplinary committees. Ultimately, the goal is to work through the problem and resolve the issue to the satisfaction of all the parties. Such a resolution may not always be possible, but when it is not, strategies to reduce the moral distress of the individuals involved should be put in place (Williams & Sudia-Robinson, 2007).

The neonatal registered nurse works in collaboration with physicians, advanced practice registered nurses, other healthcare team members, and family members to provide care that is determined to be in the best interests of the child and family. The neonatal registered nurse acknowledges the parents' role as surrogate decision-maker for the infant. The neonatal registered nurse provides the family with detailed information to enable informed decision-making and consent. Acting as an infant advocate, the neonatal registered nurse identifies potential ethical conflicts when they occur and coordinates interdisciplinary forums for discussion and resolution of these conflicts (NANN, 2010a).

Discharge Planning

The neonatal registered nurse plays an important role in partnering with the family and caregivers to coordinate the discharge of sick, medically fragile, or recovering full-term or preterm infants. Identification of the medical home should occur early in the process of discharge planning, ideally at the time of birth or as soon after birth as is reasonable for the needs of that child and family. The neonatal registered nurse must be knowledgeable about current evidence-based discharge practices. The process should be proactive and multidisciplinary and should utilize available community resources to ease the transition of the infant and family into the home environment and community. A comprehensive plan for discharge builds upon the partnership formed between the family and the healthcare team, making arrangements to assist the parents or caregivers in developing the ability to meet the infant's needs independently (Daily, Carter, & Carter, 2011). In some circumstances, the family cannot meet the needs of the infant independently. When this situation arises, identification of available resources to meet the infant's care needs is part of the discharge process.

Advocacy

Advocacy is increasingly becoming a part of the role of the neonatal nurse. Advocacy is a skill that relies upon the individual nurse's critical thinking and negotiation skills. The neonatal registered nurse is uniquely positioned to assist individual families by advocating for both the family and the infant. This advocacy can take the form of advocating for an individual infant or a group of infants with similar characteristics. For instance, an individual nurse may advocate for the development of a practice guideline to improve the care of infants experiencing pain. Additionally, advocacy may take the form of involvement in a professional organization to improve the care of infants across the country or even the world.

Quality Assurance and Evidence-Based Practice

The neonatal registered nurse utilizes evidence-based nursing practice to provide high-quality nursing care to the infant. The nurse participates in identifying potential avenues for research and quality improvement to benefit the infant and neonatal nursing care practice. The neonatal registered nurse is cognizant of current practice trends and works to improve outcomes based upon accumulated research and evidence. The neonatal registered nurse synthesizes and organizes available evidence to improve care via practice bundles and practice guidelines. Development of practice bundles and clinical practice guidelines has been shown to improve care in a variety of ways. For example, existing CDC guidelines for the prevention of catheter-related infections emphasize implementing bundled strategies and documenting compliance with all components of the bundle as a benchmark for quality assurance and performance improvement (O'Grady et al., 2011). The scrupulous implementation of central-line bundles has been widely adopted in the NICU and has resulted in a reduction in the incidence of bloodstream infections (Cooley & Grady, 2009; Taylor et al., 2011). The neonatal medical and nursing communities have worked collaboratively for years to ensure improved safety and outcomes. One example of this is the Vermont Oxford Network, a not-for-profit organization formed in the late 1980s with the goal of improving the quality and safety of care for neonatal patients around the world (Horbar, Soll, & Edwards, 2010).

Patient Safety

Medical errors affect 1 in 10 patients worldwide (WHO, 2007). The reports of the Institute of Medicine (IOM) on patient safety, quality, and errors have shaped nursing and medical care in the neonatal arena, just as they have throughout the rest of the healthcare community. The IOM emphasizes a patient-focused approach to care delivery as a solution to the "quality chasm" (IOM, 2001). The neonatal registered nurse is aware of the complexity of both the NICU environment and neonatal disease (Raju, Suresh, & Higgins, 2011). The neonatal registered nurse recognizes situations in which potential harm may befall the individual infant and takes action to prevent harm or injury. The neonatal registered nurse works to identify potential and actual causes of error and to create appropriate changes in individual practice, unit culture, and larger systems of health care (Samra, McGrath, & Rollins, 2011).

The development of policies and procedures is considerably more evidence based than in the past, with the varying strengths of evidence being critically evaluated and ranked and with evidence from systematic reviews and randomly controlled clinical trials holding more weight than less well-controlled studies or expert opinion (Ikuta & Beauman, 2011). In addition, systems to double-check medication administration and prescription have become more common. These include electronic medication administration systems, physician order entry systems, manual double-checking of medications prior to administration, and standardization of dosage concentrations. Specific challenges associated with neonatal medication administration have been delineated and recommendations published by the Institute for Safe Medication Practices (Dabliz & Levine, 2012). The neonatal nurse is aware of and employs strategies for ensuring safe medication administration.

Research

Evidence-based practice is most effective when practice decisions and guidelines are based upon solid research. Nursing research confirms existing knowledge and allows nursing practice to grow. The neonatal registered nurse recognizes the necessity of research to guide practice. The neonatal registered nurse identifies existing evidence and uses it to shape practice. The neonatal registered nurse identifies gaps in knowledge and, when possible, collaborates with nurse researchers to fill those gaps. The neonatal registered nurse critically reads and evaluates research in the literature. Multiple roles in research for the neonatal registered nurse exist. These include consumer, participant, facilitator, and investigator (Stevens & Harrison, 2007). Neonatal nursing research questions that have been explored include topics such as skin care, assessment and management of pain, developmental care, skin-to-skin care, effects of the environment, and management of breastfeeding. Many other areas of research also exist. The neonatal registered nurse identifies opportunities for utilization of nursing research. The neonatal registered nurse identifies barriers to translating research into evidence-based practice and seeks to reduce or eliminate them.

Practice Environments and Levels of Care in Neonatal Nursing

The neonatal registered nurse provides health care to the infant in a variety of settings, which may include the delivery room, newborn nursery, subacute care, acute care, chronic care, interhospital transport, home care, and infant follow-up clinics. In the hospital setting, neonatal units provide care at specific infant-acuity levels. These unit designations reflect availability of personnel, physical space, equipment, technology, and organizational resources to provide care that is required for specific neonatal populations. The definitions include minimal capabilities, functional criteria, and provider type required. Determinations of level of NICU care in this document are based on the American Academy of Pediatrics (AAP) policy statement "Levels of Neonatal Care" (2012).

- *Level I*—In Level I care, the nurse directly observes the neonate during the stabilization period after birth. The nurse monitors the low-risk newborn infant's adaptation to extra-uterine life and ideally assists in the transition of the newborn to rooming-in with the mother. The neonatal registered nurse can also practice in a mother–baby unit caring for healthy newborns. In addition, the nurse can care for physiologically stable preterm infants born at 35–37 weeks gestation. The nurse in this level of care can also stabilize infants born at less than 35 weeks gestation or who are ill until transfer to a higher level of care is provided. This level of care is an essential part of mother–infant care.

- *Level II*—In the Level II setting, often referred to as special care or transitional care, the neonatal registered nurse takes on greater responsibility for monitoring the premature newborn or the newborn who is having difficulty in adapting to extra-uterine life. The neonatal registered nurse at this level cares for observing and monitoring the premature newborn or the newborn who is having difficulty in adapting to extra-uterine life. The neonatal registered nurse at this level cares for premature infants who are born at gestation of 32 weeks or more or who weigh 1,500 grams or more at birth with problems that are expected to resolve rapidly. Full-term infants who are moderately ill or have had complications at birth are also included. Infants in Level II units are not expected to need urgent subspecialty care. The infants in this unit may require respiratory support (including assisted ventilation on an interim basis until the infant's condition improves or the infant is transferred), supplemental oxygen, intravenous therapy, specialized feeding, or time to mature prior to discharge. These units must have equipment and personnel continuously available to provide ongoing care and to address emergencies. The nurse provides the family with discharge instruction and arranges for follow-up support when the infant is discharged to home.

- *Level III*—In the Level III NICU, the neonatal registered nurse cares for the acutely ill newborn during a critical period. Expert care and knowledge are required in this highly technical and challenging environment. The nurse provides direct care for the premature or full-term infant who requires complex care. The neonatal registered nurse cares for infants requiring intensive life-support techniques, such as mechanical ventilation, nitric oxide therapy, and high-frequency ventilation. These units have continuously available personnel and equipment to provide life support for as long as is necessary. They also have access to subspecialists either on site or via prearranged telemedicine technology or telephone consultation.

- *Level IV*—In addition to all the capabilities of the Level III NICU, Level IV NICUs have the added capability to care for the most complex and critically ill infant requiring surgical repair of complex conditions, including complex congenital cardiac defects. The nurse in these units also cares for the chronically technology-dependent infant. The nurse teaches the family how to care for the child in the home setting or aids in the transition to a rehabilitation center. Many of these Level IV NICUs are also regional perinatal centers. The neonatal nurse in this setting may also be involved in facilitation and education within their referral centers.

- *Delivery Room*—The neonatal registered nurse is responsible for attending the birth of neonates deemed to be at high risk. Knowledge of common causes of infant distress at birth requiring neonatal resuscitation is essential. Every delivery should be attended by at least one individual whose sole responsibility is the care of the newborn, and this person should be skilled at initiating resuscitation. That individual or someone who is readily available should have the skills to provide a complete resuscitation, including endotracheal intubation (Kattwinkel et al., 2010).

- *Transport*—Access to tertiary care and both the technological support and staff expertise in these centers is made available through the efforts of transport teams composed of nursing, medical, and other health professionals. The neonatal registered nurse may be responsible for transporting an infant via ground or air. For those infants born acutely ill in a location without the necessary resources, the neonatal registered nurse assists the team with stabilization in preparation for transport, as well as in the actual transport to a tertiary care center. The neonatal transport nurse is responsible for assessment, stabilization, and continuous high-level care during the transfer to the tertiary care center. The neonatal registered nurse may also be responsible for transporting the stable newborn to the community-level hospital for convalescent care (Price-Douglas, Romito, & Taylor, 2010).

The care of the neonatal patient is guided by the neonatal nursing standards of practice. At all care levels, the neonatal registered nurse recognizes and demonstrates the importance of her or his role as an infant and family advocate. Training to assess minute changes in the infant's health and to observe unspoken cues and physiologic changes define this nursing practice. The neonatal registered nurse evaluates outcomes of the infant's care and revises the plan as necessary to promote wellness. Sick newborn infants require the attention of specialized, expert neonatal registered nurses at all care levels.

Education, Certification, and Roles in Neonatal Nursing

Graduation from an accredited nursing program and registered nursing licensure are required for entry into the field of neonatal nursing. Many registered nurses enter this specialty practice after having obtained pediatric or critical care nursing experience. An individualized education and orientation program supports the registered nurse in initial practice and provides the opportunity for both novice nurses and those who are new to the facility to work with an experienced preceptor. The professional neonatal registered nurse meets her or his ongoing learning needs through reading journals and books and completing professional development experiences, such as continuing education opportunities, attendance at conferences related to neonatal care, or involvement in a professional nursing organization pertinent to practice.

Neonatal registered nurses demonstrate accountability for maintaining excellence in practice through self-motivated ventures as well as collaborative efforts with other nursing colleagues, organizations, and professional associations. Maintaining core competencies within an individual's role is an expectation and can be achieved through ongoing documentation of critical thinking and psychomotor skills and within role-specific domains (National Association of Neonatal Nurse Practitioners [NANNP], 2010a, 2010b). Professional associations and organizations provide the opportunity to advocate for professional nursing, patients, and families at both the local and national levels. Participation in the specialty's certification process further demonstrates the nurse's commitment to expertise in neonatal nursing. Nurses who have developed expertise in neonatal nursing may test their proficiency through certification or specialization designation in several areas of neonatal nursing, including low-risk neonatal care, neonatal intensive care, neonatal transport, and neonatal developmental care (American Association of Critical-Care Nurses [AACN], 2012; NANN, n.d.; National Certification Corporation [NCC], 2011).

Neonatal registered nurses may seek to advance their formal education through a number of pathways, including master's, doctor of nursing practice (DNP), doctor of nursing science (DNSc), or doctor of philosophy (PhD) preparation. The advanced practice neonatal nursing role requires additional formal education in neonatal care at a minimum of master's-level preparation (NANNP, 2009). The *Consensus Model for APRN Regulation* clearly states that to be defined as an advanced practice registered nurse (APRN), the nurse must have passed an examination that "measures APRN, role and population-focused competencies and [must maintain] continued competence as evidenced by recertification in the role and population through the national certification program" (National Council of State Boards of Nursing [NCSBN], 2008, p. 6). In the neonatal setting, the APRN is an expert nurse practitioner or clinical nurse specialist who collaborates with a multidisciplinary team, including neonatologists, pediatricians, nursing staff, and the infant's family (AAP & American College of Obstetricians and Gynecologists, 2007).

The neonatal nurse practitioner (NNP) applies nursing theory and advanced knowledge and clinical training to the management of a caseload of infants, in collaboration with the neonatologist. The NNP typically is responsible for medical and nursing management of acutely ill and convalescent patients, but may also have roles in staff development, research, and the development of standards of care. Certification as an NNP is available through the NCC. Ongoing documentation of critical thinking and psychomotor skills and within role-specific domains have been developed for NNPs (NANNP, 2010a, 2010b). The neonatal clinical nurse specialist (NCNS) is responsible for fostering continuous quality improvement in neonatal nursing care. The NCNS develops and educates staff, models expert nursing practice, and applies and promotes evidence-based nursing practice. Doctorally prepared neonatal nurses may focus on conducting research to test caregiving practices and develop theory, with varying degrees of clinically focused clinical practice. Both master's- and doctorally prepared APRNs can teach neonatal nursing in the college or hospital setting (NANN, 2009a).

Future Considerations

Neonatology is a rapidly evolving field, and each year brings forth substantial research and recommendations for practice changes. Genetic testing and research related to genetic therapy will increasingly influence neonatal care (National Human Genome Project, 2010). Direct fetal treatment procedures, which merge the roles of delivery room nurse, surgical nurse, and neonatal nurse, have the potential for creating new neonatal patient populations. These populations will have new needs, some of which can be anticipated and some of which will not be expected.

Through evaluation of ongoing research, the neonatal registered nurse strives to develop and implement evidence-based practice. Increased use of electronic medical records will increase the ability to "mine" data and make it possible to more efficiently assess areas for improving care. Electronic medical records and automation of devices to allow synchronization of data to the medical record will result in changes in care delivery and work flow. Electronic records will also assist in improving safety with decision support modules and clinical warnings. Collaborative projects involving nursing and medicine, as well as networks to evaluate outcomes, will offer opportunities to improve care. Quality improvement activity is becoming the norm in NICUs around the country. Pay-for-performance has been implemented in some areas of adult care already and will likely come to the neonatal world in the future (Profit, Zupancic, Gould, & Petersen, 2007). The neonatal registered nurse has the opportunity to enact change through appraisal of research, which will enable the profession to grow and establish professional credibility (Stevens & Harrison, 2007).

Advances in both prenatal and perinatal treatment (e.g., infertility assistance or fetal treatment) have altered the context of neonatal care practice. Low-birthweight and premature infants account for more than 8% and 12% of births, respectively (CDC, 2006). Increased numbers of multigestation pregnancies, late-preterm infants, and medically fragile infants have increased the demand for care providers versed in the care of these patients. Extremely premature and other compromised infants are surviving to discharge with increased levels of complex needs, reinforcing the need for neonatal registered nurses who can also provide care for the newborn in the home. The nurse in this role may provide or direct technically advanced care and follow-up care coordination. The expanding roles for neonatal registered nurses have created a national need at all provider levels.

The neonatal registered nurse's role will change as new technology and treatments are developed. Improvements in care outcomes must be evaluated in light of cost, equitability, and feasibility. Ethical decision-making will continue to be an important part of the neonatal registered nurse's daily work and will likely become more complex. As NICU cases escalate in acuity and complexity, and as the issues of payment for services are affected by healthcare reform, the stress that all healthcare providers experience may increase. It is important that neonatal registered nurses be supported in this stressful environment. Recruitment and retention of nursing staff and support of new graduates entering the profession are crucial for the advancement and survival of the profession and neonatal nursing specialty.

Standards of Neonatal Nursing Practice

Standards of Practice for Neonatal Nursing

Standard 1. Assessment

The neonatal registered nurse collects comprehensive data pertinent to the infant's health and/or the family situation.

COMPETENCIES

The neonatal registered nurse:

- Collects comprehensive data including, but not limited to, physical, functional, psychosocial, developmental, emotional, mental, sexual, cultural, age-related, environmental, spiritual/transpersonal, and economic assessments in a systematic and ongoing process while honoring the uniqueness of the infant and the family.

- Elicits the family's values, preferences, expressed needs, and knowledge of the healthcare situation.

- Involves the parents of the infant, family/support system, other healthcare providers, and environment, as appropriate, in holistic data collection.

- Identifies barriers (psychosocial, financial, cultural, etc.) to effective communication and makes appropriate adaptations.

- Recognizes the impact of personal attitudes, values, and beliefs when assessing infants and their families with diverse backgrounds or situations.

- Assesses family dynamics and their impact on the infant's health and wellness.

- Prioritizes data collection activities based on the infant's immediate condition or on the anticipated developmental and health needs of the infant.

- Uses appropriate evidence-based assessment techniques and instruments and tools.

- Synthesizes available data, information, and knowledge relevant to the situation to identify patterns and variances.

- Documents relevant data in a retrievable format.

- Applies ethical, legal, and privacy guidelines and policies to the collection, maintenance, use, and dissemination of data and information.

- Recognizes the parents as the authority on their infant's health and honors their role as surrogate decision-makers in regard to the care of the infant.

ADDITIONAL COMPETENCIES FOR THE ADVANCED PRACTICE REGISTERED NURSE

The advanced practice registered nurse:

- Initiates and interprets diagnostic tests and procedures relevant to the infant's current status.

- Assesses the effect of interactions among individuals, family, community, and social systems on health, illness, and development.

Standard 2. Diagnosis

The neonatal registered nurse analyzes the assessment data to determine the diagnosis or issue.

COMPETENCIES

The neonatal registered nurse:

- Derives diagnoses using assessment data that reflect the infant's current clinical condition and potential outcomes for that situation.

- Revises diagnoses regularly, based on integration of current and relevant historical data.

- Validates diagnoses with the infant's family and other healthcare providers when possible and appropriate.

- Identifies actual and potential risks to the infant's health and safety, including:

  - The infant's identified or potential physiologic and developmental problems

  - The infant's integration into the family during the period of hospitalization and after discharge

  - The support, educational, and developmental needs of the family

  - Any present or potential environmental, systematic problems or barriers to health.

- Uses standardized classification systems and clinical decision support tools, when available, in identifying diagnoses.

- Documents diagnoses and issues in a manner that facilitates the expected outcomes and the plan of care.

ADDITIONAL COMPETENCIES FOR THE ADVANCED PRACTICE REGISTERED NURSE

The advanced practice registered nurse:

- Systematically compares and contrasts clinical findings and data, including normal and abnormal variations, within a developmental context when formulating a differential diagnosis.

- Utilizes complex data and information obtained during review of history, interview, examination, and diagnostic procedures in identifying diagnoses.

- Assists staff in developing and maintaining competency in the diagnostic process.

Standard 3. Outcomes Identification

The neonatal registered nurse identifies expected outcomes for a plan individualized to the infant or the situation.

COMPETENCIES

The neonatal registered nurse:

- Involves the parents, and if the parents desire, the extended family, significant others, and other healthcare providers to formulate expected outcomes whenever possible and appropriate.

- Uses culturally appropriate strategies to identify expected outcomes for each infant and family unit.

- Considers associated risks, benefits, costs, current scientific evidence, expected trajectory for the infant/child, family structure and expectations, and clinical resources when formulating expected outcomes.

- Defines expected outcomes in terms of the infant, family values, ethical considerations, environment, or situation in respect to associated risks, benefits, costs, and current scientific evidence.

- Includes a time estimate for the attainment of expected outcomes.

- Develops expected outcomes that provide direction for continuity of care, both during the acute hospitalization and as the infant transitions back into the community.

- Modifies expected outcomes based on changes in the status of the infant or evaluation of the situation.

- Documents expected outcomes as measurable goals.

ADDITIONAL COMPETENCIES FOR THE ADVANCED PRACTICE REGISTERED NURSE

The advanced practice registered nurse:

- Identifies expected outcomes that incorporate scientific evidence and are achievable through implementation of evidence-based practices.

- Identifies expected outcomes that incorporate cost and clinical effectiveness, family satisfaction, and continuity and consistency of care among providers.

- Differentiates outcomes that require process interventions at the infant or family level from those that require system-level interventions.

Standard 4. Planning

The neonatal registered nurse develops a plan of care that prescribes interventions to attain expected outcomes.

COMPETENCIES

The neonatal registered nurse:

- Uses appropriate physiologic, developmental, and social data and diagnoses to develop an individualized plan of care for the infant.

- Develops a plan that is individualized to the infant and family, including, but not limited to, the family's values, beliefs, spiritual and health practices, preferences, choices, coping style, family developmental level, culture, environment, and available technology.

- Develops the plan in partnership with the family and other healthcare providers whenever appropriate.

- Includes strategies in the plan of care that address each identified diagnosis or issue and promote or restore health; prevent illness, injury, and disease; alleviate suffering; and provide supportive and/or palliative care when needed.

- Ensures that the plan is a continuous and dynamic process that addresses the needs of the infant and incorporates an implementation pathway or timeline.

- Develops a plan that incorporates the family in caregiving and reflects priorities of the family, the infant, and the healthcare team.

- Utilizes the plan to provide direction to other members of the healthcare team.

- Defines the plan to reflect current statutes, rules and regulations, and practice standards.

- Integrates current evidence-based practice, trends, and research in care planning.

- Considers the economic impact of the plan on the family, caregivers, and other affected parties.

- Documents the plan of care in a manner that uses standardized language and recognized terminology and is understood by all participants.

- Includes strategies that optimize health, wholeness, growth, and development.

- Organizes, integrates, and plans care with consideration for the infant's stage of development.

- Provides a safe atmosphere for the nurse and family to explore traditional, potential, and alternative options for care.

- Modifies the plan based on ongoing assessment of the infant's response and other outcome indicators.

ADDITIONAL COMPETENCIES FOR THE ADVANCED PRACTICE REGISTERED NURSE

The advanced practice registered nurse:

- Identifies assessment strategies, diagnostic strategies, and therapeutic and developmental interventions within the plan that reflect current evidence, including data, research, literature, and expert clinical knowledge.

- Selects or designs strategies to meet the multifaceted needs of special-care infants and their families as complex healthcare consumers.

- Includes the synthesis of family or caregiver values and beliefs regarding nursing and medical therapies within the plan.

- Leads the design and development of intraprofessional and interprofessional processes to address the situation or issue.

- Actively participates in the development and continuous improvement of systems that support the planning process.

Standard 5. Implementation

The neonatal registered nurse implements the identified plan.

COMPETENCIES

The neonatal registered nurse:

- In partnership with the family, significant others, and other caregivers, implements the plan in a safe, timely, and realistic manner.

- Demonstrates caring behaviors toward infants and families as healthcare consumers.

- Utilizes technology to measure, record, and retrieve healthcare consumer data, implement the nursing process, and enhance nursing practice.

- Utilizes evidence-based knowledge, treatments, and strategies specific to the issue, problem, diagnosis, or trend.

- Provides holistic care that addresses the needs of infants and their families with diverse socioeconomic, cultural, and developmental needs.

- Advocates for health care that is sensitive to the needs of infants and their families, with particular emphasis on the needs of diverse populations and family structures.

- Applies appropriate knowledge of major health problems and their sequelae in implementing the plan of care.

- Applies healthcare technologies to optimize access and outcomes for infants.

- Utilizes community resources when appropriate to maximize health and developmental outcomes.

- Collaborates with healthcare providers from diverse backgrounds and the family to implement the plan.

- Accommodates different styles of communication used by healthcare consumers, families, and healthcare providers.

- Integrates traditional and complementary healthcare practices as appropriate.

- Implements the plan of care in a manner that is timely and systematic, in accordance with patient safety goals.

- Promotes the family's capacity for an optimal level of participation and problem-solving, honoring the decision-making process of the family when appropriate.

- Documents implementation and any modifications or omissions of the identified plan.

- Organizes interventions to provide an environment that supports the family's and infant's physical and developmental well-being.

ADDITIONAL COMPETENCIES FOR THE ADVANCED PRACTICE REGISTERED NURSE

The advanced practice registered nurse:

- Facilitates utilization of systems, organizations, and community resources to develop the plan.

- Supports collaboration with nursing colleagues and other disciplines to implement and update the interprofessional plan.

- Incorporates new knowledge and strategies to initiate change if desired outcomes are not achieved.

- Assumes responsibility for safe and efficient implementation of the plan of care.

- Uses advanced communication skills to promote relationships between nurses and families, to provide a context for open discussion of the infant's and family's experiences, and to improve patient safety and outcomes.

- Actively participates in the development and continuous improvement of systems that support implementation of the plan of care.

Standard 5A. Coordination of Care

The neonatal registered nurse coordinates care delivery.

COMPETENCIES

The neonatal registered nurse:

- Coordinates implementation of the plan.

- Manages care to meet the special needs of the vulnerable infant in order to maximize growth, development, and quality of life.

- Assists the family and care providers to recognize viable options and alternatives.

- Communicates with the family and community resources during transitions in care.

- Advocates for the delivery of dignified and humane care by the interprofessional team.

- Initiates referrals, including provisions for continuity of care, as needed.

- Documents the coordination of the plans.

ADDITIONAL COMPETENCIES FOR THE ADVANCED PRACTICE REGISTERED NURSE

The advanced practice registered nurse:

- Provides leadership in the coordination of multidisciplinary healthcare and community resources to provide integrated delivery of family-centered care.

- Synthesizes data and information to prescribe necessary system and community support measures, including meeting educational needs of the family and making environmental modifications to the home.

Standard 5B. Health Teaching and Health Promotion

The neonatal registered nurse employs strategies to promote health and a safe environment.

COMPETENCIES

The neonatal registered nurse:

- Provides the family or caregiver with health teaching that addresses such topics as healthy lifestyle, risk-reduction behaviors, developmental needs, and anticipatory infant care and safety.

- Uses health promotion and health teaching methods, including information technologies, appropriate to the situation, setting, and parent's or caregiver's values, beliefs, health practices, developmental level, learning needs, readiness and ability to learn, language preference, spirituality, culture, and socioeconomic status.

- Seeks opportunities for feedback and evaluation of the effectiveness of the strategies used.

- Provides the family or caregiver with information about intended effects and potential adverse effects of proposed therapies.

ADDITIONAL COMPETENCIES FOR THE ADVANCED PRACTICE REGISTERED NURSE

The advanced practice registered nurse:

- Synthesizes empirical evidence on risk behaviors, learning theories, behavioral change theories, motivational theories, epidemiology, and other frameworks when designing health information and education for families or caregivers.

- Conducts individualized health teaching and counseling, considering research recommendations on comparative effectiveness.

- Designs health information and family or caregiver education appropriate to their developmental level, learning needs, readiness to learn, and cultural values and beliefs.

- Evaluates health information resources, such as those on the Internet, within the area of practice for accuracy, reliability, readability, and comprehensibility to help patients access high-quality health information.

- Engages consumer alliances and advocacy groups, as appropriate, in health teaching and health promotion activities.

- Provides anticipatory guidance to individuals, families, groups, and communities to promote health and prevent or reduce the risk of health problems.

Standard 5C. Consultation

The advanced practice registered nurse provides consultation to influence the identified plan, enhance the abilities of others, and effect change.

COMPETENCIES FOR THE ADVANCED
PRACTICE REGISTERED NURSE:
The advanced practice registered nurse:

- Synthesizes clinical data, information, theoretical frameworks, and evidence when providing consultation.

- Facilitates the effectiveness of a consultation by involving the family, caregiver, and stakeholders in decision-making and negotiating role responsibilities.

- Communicates consultation recommendations to facilitate change.

- Seeks and provides appropriate interprofessional consultation to improve outcomes.

Standard 5D. Prescriptive Authority and Treatment

The advanced practice registered nurse uses prescriptive authority, procedures, referrals, treatments, and therapies in accordance with state and federal laws and regulations.

**COMPETENCIES FOR THE ADVANCED
PRACTICE REGISTERED NURSE**

The advanced practice registered nurse:

- Prescribes evidence-based treatments, therapies, and procedures considering the infant's comprehensive healthcare needs.

- Prescribes pharmacologic agents based on a current knowledge of neonatal pharmacology and physiology.

- Prescribes specific pharmacologic agents and/or treatments based on clinical indicators, the infant's status and needs, and the results of diagnostic and laboratory tests.

- Evaluates therapeutic and potential adverse effects of pharmacologic and nonpharmacologic treatments.

- Provides families with information about intended effects and potential adverse effects of proposed prescriptive therapies.

- Provides information about costs, alternative treatments, and procedures, as appropriate.

- Evaluates and incorporates alternative therapy into education and practice when appropriate.

Standard 6. Evaluation

The neonatal registered nurse evaluates progress toward attainment of goals.

COMPETENCIES

The neonatal registered nurse:

- Conducts a systematic, ongoing, and criterion-based evaluation of outcomes in relationship to the structures and processes prescribed by the plan of care and the associated timeline.

- Collaborates with the family and all others involved in the care or situation in the evaluation process.

- Evaluates, in partnership with the family, the effectiveness of the planned strategies in relation to attainment of the expected outcomes.

- Uses ongoing assessment data and the priorities of the family and the healthcare team to revise the diagnoses, outcomes, plan, and implementation as needed.

- Disseminates the results to the healthcare consumer, family, and others involved, in accordance with federal and state laws.

- Participates in assessing and ensuring the responsible and appropriate use of interventions so as to minimize unwarranted or unwanted treatment and suffering.

- Documents the results of the evaluation.

ADDITIONAL COMPETENCIES FOR THE ADVANCED PRACTICE REGISTERED NURSE

The advanced practice registered nurse:

- Evaluates the accuracy of the diagnosis and effectiveness of the interventions and other variables in relationship to the infant's and family's attainment of expected outcomes.

- Synthesizes the results of the evaluation to determine the effect of the plan on healthcare consumers, families, groups, communities, and institutions.

- Adapts the plan of care for the anticipated course of treatment based on evaluation of response.

- Uses the results of the evaluation to make or recommend process or structural changes, including policy, procedure, or protocol revision, as appropriate.

Standards of Professional Performance for Neonatal Nursing

Standard 7. Ethics

The neonatal registered nurse practices ethically.

COMPETENCIES

The neonatal registered nurse:

- Uses *Code of Ethics for Nurses with Interpretive Statements* (ANA, 2001) to guide and inform practice.

- Delivers care in a manner that preserves and protects infant and family autonomy, dignity, rights, values, and beliefs.

- Recognizes the centrality of the family as core members of any healthcare team.

- Upholds infant and family confidentiality within legal and regulatory parameters.

- Assists the family in self-determination and informed decision-making.

- Maintains a therapeutic and professional family–nurse relationship with appropriate professional role boundaries.

- Contributes to resolving ethical issues involving familes, colleagues, community groups, systems, and other stakeholders.

- Takes appropriate action regarding instances of illegal, unethical, or inappropriate behavior that can endanger or jeopardize the best interests of the infant, family, or situation.

- Speaks up when appropriate to question healthcare practice and intervenes when necessary to promote safety and quality improvement.

- Advocates for equitable care and assists the family in developing skills to become advocates for their own infant.

**ADDITIONAL COMPETENCIES FOR THE ADVANCED
PRACTICE REGISTERED NURSE**

The advanced practice registered nurse:

- Participates in interprofessional teams that address ethical risks, benefits, and outcomes.

- Provides information on the risks, benefits, and outcomes of healthcare regimens to allow informed decision-making by the family, including informed consent and informed refusal.

- Advocates for and counsels members of the interprofessional team in dealing with ethical issues.

Standard 8. Education

The neonatal registered nurse acquires knowledge and competence that reflect current neonatal nursing practice.

COMPETENCIES

The neonatal registered nurse:

- Participates in ongoing educational activities related to clinical and theoretical knowledge and professional issues.

- Demonstrates a commitment to lifelong learning through self-reflection and inquiry to address learning and personal growth needs.

- Seeks experiences that reflect current practice to maintain knowledge, skills, abilities, and judgment in clinical practice or role performance.

- Acquires knowledge and skills appropriate to the neonatal specialty area, practice setting, role, and learner diversity.

- Seeks formal and independent learning experiences to develop and maintain clinical and professional skills and knowledge.

- Identifies learning needs based on nursing knowledge, the various roles the nurse may assume, and the changing needs of the population.

- Participates in formal or informal consultations to address issues in nursing practice as an application of education and knowledge base.

- Shares educational findings, experiences, and ideas with peers.

- Contributes to a work environment that is conducive to the education of healthcare professionals.

- Maintains professional records that provide evidence of competency and lifelong learning.

ADDITIONAL COMPETENCIES FOR THE ADVANCED PRACTICE REGISTERED NURSE

The advanced practice registered nurse:

- Uses current healthcare research findings and other evidence to expand clinical knowledge, skills, abilities, and judgment to enhance role performance and increase knowledge of professional issues.

Standard 9. Evidence-Based Practice and Research

The neonatal registered nurse integrates evidence and research findings into practice.

COMPETENCIES

The neonatal registered nurse:

- Utilizes current evidence-based nursing knowledge, including research findings, to develop the plan of care and guide practice decisions.

- Incorporates evidence when initiating changes in nursing practice.

- Participates, as appropriate to educational level and position, in the development of evidence-based practice through research activities. These activities may include:

  - Identification of clinical problems pertinent to neonatal nursing care.

  - Participation in all aspects of the research process, as appropriate, including data collection.

  - Participation in unit, organizational, community, or global research activities.

  - Dissemination of evidence-based practice and research information and findings with peers and others.

  - Conduct of research, including use of ethical principles.

  - Critique of research for application to neonatal practice.

  - Use of evidence-based practice and research findings in the development of policies, procedures, and practice guidelines for neonatal care.

  - Use of evidence-based practice and research findings to advance the state of nursing science in the care of infants and their families.

- Shares personal or third-party research findings with colleagues and peers.

ADDITIONAL COMPETENCIES FOR THE ADVANCED PRACTICE REGISTERED NURSE

The advanced practice registered nurse:

- Contributes to nursing knowledge by conducting or synthesizing research and other evidence that discovers, examines, and evaluates current practice, knowledge, theories, criteria, and creative approaches to improve neonatal practice and outcomes.

- Formally disseminates research findings through activities such as presentations, publications, consultation, and journal clubs.

- Promotes a climate of research and clinical inquiry.

Standard 10. Quality of Practice

The neonatal registered nurse contributes to quality nursing practice.

COMPETENCIES

The neonatal registered nurse:

- Demonstrates quality by documenting the application of the nursing process in a responsible, accountable, and ethical manner.

- Uses creativity and innovation to enhance nursing care, adapting new innovations to the NICU environment.

- Works collaboratively with the healthcare team to integrate scientific research and evidence-based practice.

- Obtains and maintains professional requirements for licensure and employment based upon the individual role, state licensure requirements, and employer.

- Participates in quality improvement activities appropriate to the nurse's education and role. Such activities may include:

    - Identifying aspects of practice important for quality monitoring and improvement.

    - Using indicators developed to monitor the quality, safety, and effectiveness of nursing practice.

    - Collecting data to monitor the quality and effectiveness of nursing practice.

    - Analyzing quality data to identify opportunities for improving nursing practice and care delivery.

    - Formulating recommendations to improve nursing practice or outcomes.

    - Implementing activities to enhance the quality of nursing practice.

    - Developing, implementing, and evaluating policies, procedures, and guidelines to improve the quality of practice.

- Participating on or leading interprofessional teams to evaluate care of the neonate or services provided to the neonate.

- Participating in or leading efforts to minimize costs and unnecessary duplication.

- Identifying problems that occur in day-to-day work flow in the NICU in order to correct process inefficiencies.

- Analyzing factors related to quality, safety, and effectiveness.

- Analyzing organizational systems for barriers to high-quality neonatal outcomes.

- Implementing processes to remove or decrease barriers within organizational systems.

ADDITIONAL COMPETENCIES FOR THE ADVANCED PRACTICE REGISTERED NURSE

The advanced practice registered nurse:

- Provides leadership in the design and implementation of quality improvement activities.

- Designs innovations to effect change in practice and improve neonatal outcomes.

- Evaluates the neonatal environment and quality of nursing care rendered in relation to existing evidence.

- Identifies opportunities for the generation and use of research and evidence.

- Obtains and maintains professional certification if available in the area of expertise.

- Applies the results of quality improvement activities to initiate changes in nursing practice and neonatal nursing or in the healthcare delivery system.

Standard 11. Communication

The neonatal registered nurse communicates effectively in all areas of practice, using a variety of formats.

COMPETENCIES

The neonatal registered nurse:

- Assesses communication format preferences of healthcare consumers, families, and colleagues.

- Assesses her or his own communication skills in encounters with healthcare consumers, families, and colleagues.

- Seeks continuous improvement of her or his own communication and conflict resolution skills.

- Conveys information to healthcare consumers, families, the NICU team, and others in communication formats that promote accuracy.

- Questions the rationale supporting care processes and decisions when they do not appear to be in the best interest of the neonate.

- Discloses to the appropriate level any observations or concerns related to hazards or errors in delivery of care or the neonatal practice environment.

- Maintains clear, effective communication with other members of the healthcare team to minimize risks associated with handoff and transition in care delivery.

- Contributes her or his own professional perspective in discussions with the neonatal team.

Standard 12. Leadership

The neonatal registered nurse demonstrates leadership in the professional practice setting and the profession.

COMPETENCIES

The neonatal registered nurse:

- Oversees the nursing care given by others while retaining accountability for the quality of care given to the infant and family.

- Abides by the vision, the associated goals, and plan of care to implement and measure the progress of an individual infant or within the context of the healthcare organization.

- Demonstrates a commitment to continuous lifelong learning and education for self and others.

- Mentors colleagues for the advancement of nursing practice, the profession, and quality health care.

- Treats colleagues with respect, trust, and dignity.

- Employs therapeutic communication and conflict resolution skills.

- Actively participates in professional organizations.

- Communicates effectively with the family and colleagues.

- Seeks ways to advance nursing autonomy and accountability.

- Participates in efforts to influence healthcare policy involving infants, families, and the profession.

ADDITIONAL COMPETENCIES FOR THE ADVANCED PRACTICE REGISTERED NURSE

The advanced practice registered nurse:

- Influences decision-making bodies to improve the professional practice environment and infant outcomes.

- Provides direction to enhance the effectiveness of the interprofessional team.

- Promotes advanced practice nursing and role development by interpreting the role of advanced practice nursing for families and others.

- Models expert practice to interprofessional team members.

- Mentors colleagues in the acquisition of clinical knowledge, skills, abilities, and judgment.

Standard 13. Collaboration

The neonatal registered nurse collaborates with the family, caregivers, and others in the conduct of nursing practice.

COMPETENCIES

The neonatal registered nurse:

- Partners with others to effect change and generate positive outcomes through the sharing of knowledge of the infant, family, and situation.

- Communicates with the family and healthcare providers regarding care and the nurse's role in the provision of that care.

- Promotes conflict management and engagement.

- Participates in building consensus or resolving conflict in the context of infant care.

- Applies group process and negotiation techniques with families and colleagues.

- Adheres to standards and applicable codes of conduct that govern behavior among peers and colleagues to create a work environment promoting cooperation, respect, and trust.

- Cooperates in creating a documented plan focused on outcomes and decisions related to care and delivery of services that indicates communication with healthcare consumers, families, and others.

- Engages in teamwork and team-building processes.

- Contributes to an environment that is conducive to clinical education of students and healthcare trainees, as appropriate.

ADDITIONAL COMPETENCIES FOR THE ADVANCED PRACTICE REGISTERED NURSE

The advanced practice registered nurse:

- Partners with other disciplines to enhance infant care and outcomes through interprofessional activities, such as education, consultation, management, technological development, or research opportunities.

- Invites the contribution of the family and team members in order to achieve optimal outcomes.

- Leads in establishing, improving, and sustaining collaborative relationships to achieve safe, high-quality health care.

- Documents plans of care, rationales for changes in the plans, and collaborative discussions to improve infant care and outcomes.

- Models expert practice to the interdisciplinary team and mentors other nurses and colleagues as appropriate.

Standard 14. Professional Practice Evaluation

The neonatal registered nurse evaluates her or his own nursing practice in relation to professional practice standards and guidelines, relevant statutes, rules, and regulations.

COMPETENCIES

The neonatal registered nurse:

- Ensures that her or his practice conforms with current practice standards, guidelines, statutes, rules, and regulations.

- Provides age-appropriate and developmentally appropriate care in a culturally and ethnically sensitive manner.

- Engages in self-evaluation of practice on a regular basis, identifying areas of strength as well as areas in which professional development would be beneficial.

- Obtains informal feedback regarding her or his own practice from patients' families, peers, professional colleagues, and others on an ongoing basis for the purpose of professional development.

- Participates in peer review as appropriate.

- Takes action to achieve professional goals identified during the evaluation process.

- Demonstrates knowledge of current professional practice standards, laws, and regulations.

- Provides the evidence for practice decisions and actions as part of the informal and formal evaluation processes.

- Interacts with peers and colleagues to enhance her or his own professional nursing practice or role performance.

- Provides peers with formal or informal constructive feedback regarding their practice or role performance.

**ADDITIONAL COMPETENCIES FOR THE ADVANCED
PRACTICE REGISTERED NURSE**

The advanced practice registered nurse:

- Engages in a formal process seeking feedback regarding her or his own practice from infants' families, peers, professional colleagues, and others.

Standard 15. Resource Utilization

The neonatal registered nurse utilizes appropriate resources to plan and provide nursing services that are safe, effective, and financially responsible.

COMPETENCIES

The neonatal registered nurse:

- Assesses the individual infant and family care needs and resources available to achieve desired outcomes.

- Identifies and allocates resources based on the infant and family care needs, potential for harm, complexity of the task, and desired outcome.

- Delegates elements of care to appropriate healthcare workers in accordance with any applicable legal or policy parameters or principles.

- Advocates for the design and implementation of technology that enhances nursing practice and healthcare delivery.

- Modifies practice when necessary to promote a positive interface between the infant's family, care providers, and technology.

- Assists the infant's family in identifying and securing appropriate and available services to address needs across the healthcare continuum.

- Identifies and evaluates the cost and benefit of available resources and assists the infant's family in understanding costs, risk, and benefits of treatment and care.

ADDITIONAL COMPETENCIES FOR THE ADVANCED PRACTICE REGISTERED NURSE

The advanced practice registered nurse:

- Utilizes organizational and community resources to formulate interprofessional plans of care.

- In managing problems that arise when caring for infants, develops innovative solutions that address effective resource utilization and maintenance of quality.

- Develops evaluation strategies to demonstrate cost effectiveness, cost benefit, and efficiency factors associated with nursing practice.

Standard 16. Environmental Health

The neonatal registered nurse practices in an environmentally safe and healthy manner.

COMPETENCIES

The neonatal registered nurse:

- Attains knowledge of environmental health concepts, such as implementation of environmental health strategies.

- Promotes a practice environment that reduces environmental health risks of workers, infants, and families.

- Assesses the practice environment for factors such as sound, odor, noise, light, and potentially toxic products that negatively affect health, particularly for the vulnerable population of premature and sick infants.

- Advocates for the judicious and appropriate use of products used in health care.

- Communicates environmental health risks and exposure reduction strategies to families, colleagues, interdisciplinary teams, and communities.

- Utilizes scientific evidence to determine whether a product or treatment is a potential environmental threat.

- Participates in strategies to promote healthy communities.

ADDITIONAL COMPETENCIES FOR THE ADVANCED PRACTICE REGISTERED NURSE

The advanced practice registered nurse:

- Creates partnerships that promote sustainable environmental health policies and conditions.

- Analyzes the impact of social, political, and economic influences upon the environment and human health exposures.

- Critically evaluates the manner in which environmental health issues are presented by the popular media.

- Advocates for implementation of environmental principles in nursing practice.

- Supports nurses in advocating for and implementing environmental principles in nursing practice.

Glossary

Chronic lung disease (CLD). A long-term respiratory condition that is acquired by premature infants who are exposed to supplemental oxygen, mechanical ventilation, or both.

Developmental care. A strategy used in the neonatal intensive care unit to reduce stress and promote rest and comfort in infants who are ill. Key components of developmental care include appropriate positioning, clustering of care, provision of an appropriate healing environment, parental interaction, protection of sleep, and assessment of pain and stress.

Low-birth-weight infant. Infant born at a birth weight of less than 2,500 grams.

Neonatal. Related to the period of time encompassing the first month of life.

Neonatal intensive care unit (NICU). An intensive care unit designed specifically to meet the needs of infants who are born prematurely or who are seriously ill.

Neutral thermal environment. An environment created by any method that maintains normal body temperature and minimizes oxygen consumption and caloric expenditure.

Perinatal. Related to the period of time immediately before and after birth. Commonly, this period begins at the 20th week of pregnancy and extends through the 4th week after delivery.

Premature (preterm) infant. An infant born before the completion of the 37th week of pregnancy.

Respiratory distress syndrome (RDS). An acute lung disease found in newborns (and more commonly in infants born prematurely) that is caused mainly by a deficiency in surfactant, which prevents the collapse of the infants' alveoli, or air sacs.

Skin-to-skin care. Also known as *kangaroo care.* A care practice that uses skin-to-skin contact between the infant and a parent, most commonly with the infant being held on the parent's chest.

References

American Academy of Pediatrics & American College of Obstetricians and Gynecologists. (2007). *Guidelines for perinatal care* (6th ed.). Elk Grove Village, IL: American Academy of Pediatrics.

American Academy of Pediatrics, Committee on the Fetus and Newborn. (2012). Policy statement: Levels of neonatal care. *Pediatrics, 130*(3), 587–597. (doi: 10.1542/peds.2012–1999) Retrieved from http://pediatrics .aappublications.org/content/130/3/587.full

American Association of Critical-Care Nurses (2012). *Certification.* Retrieved from http://www.aacn.org/DM/MainPages/CertificationHome.aspx

American Nurses Association. (2001). *Code of ethics for nurses with interpretive statements.* Washington, DC: American Nurses Publishing.

American Nurses Association. (2010a). *Nursing: Scope and standards of practice* (2nd ed.). Silver Spring, MD: Author.

American Nurses Association. (2010b). *Nursing's social policy statement: The essence of the profession.* Silver Spring, MD: Author.

Barksdale, D. J. (2009). Provider factors affecting adherence: Cultural competency and sensitivity. *Ethnicity & Disease, 19*(4, Suppl. 5), S5-3–S5-7.

Catlin, A. (2009). Five incredible babies, five paradigm cases that greatly influenced neonatal ethics: What do their parents say today? *Advances in Neonatal Care, 9*(6), 287–292.

Centers for Disease Control and Prevention. (2006). *Birthweight and gestation.* Retrieved from http://www.cdc.gov

Cooley, K., & Grady, S. (2009). Minimizing catheter-related bloodstream infections. *Advances in Neonatal Care, 9*(5), 209–225.

Coughlin, M. E. (2011). *Age-appropriate care of the premature and critically ill hospitalized infant: Guideline for practice.* Glenview, IL: National Association of Neonatal Nurses. Retrieved from http://www.nann.org/uploads/Age-Appropriate_Care-FINAL_11-01-11.pdf

Dabliz, R., & Levine, S. (2012). Medication safety in neonates. *American Journal of Perinatology, 29*(1), 49–56.

Daily, D. K., Carter, A., & Carter, B. S. (2011). Discharge planning and follow-up of the neonatal intensive care unit infant. In S. Gardner, B. Carter, M. Enzman-Hines, & J. Hernandez (Eds.), *Neonatal intensive care* (7th ed., pp. 938–961). St. Louis, MO: Mosby Elsevier.

Devaskar, S. U., & Calkins, K. (2011). Developmental origins of adult health and disease. In R. J. Martin, A. A. Fanaroff, & M. C. Walsh (Eds.), *Neonatal-perinatal medicine: Diseases of the fetus and infant* (pp. 229–241). St. Louis, MO: Elsevier.

Gardner, S., Carter, B., Enzman-Hines, M., & Hernandez, J. (Eds.). (2011). *Neonatal intensive care* (7th ed.). St. Louis, MO: Mosby Elsevier.

Gardner, S. L., & Goldson, E. (2011). The neonate and the environment: Impact on development. In S. Gardner, B. Carter, M. Enzman-Hines, & J. Hernandez (Eds.), *Neonatal intensive care* (7th ed., pp. 270–331). St. Louis, MO: Mosby Elsevier.

Griffin, T. (2006). Family-centered care in the NICU. *Journal of Perinatal & Neonatal Nursing, 20*(1), 98–102.

Horbar, J. D., Soll, R. F., & Edwards, W. H. (2010). The Vermont Oxford Network: A community of practice. *Clinics in Perinatology, 37*(1), 29–47.

Ikuta, L. M., & Beauman, S. S. (Eds). (2011). *Policies, procedures, and competencies for neonatal nursing care.* Glenview, IL: National Association of Neonatal Nurses.

Institute of Medicine. (2001). *Crossing the quality chasm: A new health system for the 21st century.* Washington, DC: National Academy Press.

Kattwinkel, J., Perlman, J. M., Aziz, K., Colby, C., Fairchild, K., Gallagher, J., . . . & Zaichkin, J. (2010). Special report—Neonatal resuscitation: 2010 American Heart Association guidelines for cardiopulmonary resuscitation and emergency cardiovascular care. *Pediatrics, 126*(5), e1400–1413. Retrieved from http://pediatrics.aappublications.org/content/126/5/ e1400.full.pdf.

Kavanaugh, K., & Wheeler, S. R. (2007). When a baby dies: Caring for bereaved families. In C. Kenner & J. W. Lott (Eds.), *Comprehensive neonatal care: An interdisciplinary approach* (4th ed., pp. 522–542). St. Louis, MO: Saunders Elsevier.

Kenner, C., & McGrath, J. M. (Eds.). (2010). *Developmental care of newborns and infants: A guide for health professionals* (2nd ed.). Glenview, IL: National Association of Neonatal Nurses.

Kenner, C., & Sudia-Robinson, T. (2007). Palliative and end-of-life care. In C. Kenner & J. W. Lott (Eds.), *Comprehensive neonatal care: An interdisciplinary approach* (4th ed., pp. 510–521). St. Louis, MO: Saunders Elsevier.

March of Dimes. (2010). *Perinatal overview*. Retrieved from http://www .marchofdimes.com

Mathews, T. J., & MacDorman, M. F. (2008). *Infant mortality statistics from the 2005 period linked birth/infant death data set*. Retrieved from http:// www.cdc.gov/nchs/data/nvsr/nvsr57/nvsr57_02.pdf

National Association of Neonatal Nurse Practitioners. (2009). *Requirements for advanced neonatal nursing practice in neonatal intensive care units* [Position Statement #3042]. Retrieved from http://www.nann.org /pdf/10req_annp.pdf

National Association of Neonatal Nurse Practitioners. (2010a). *Competencies and orientation tool kit for neonatal nurse practitioners*. Glenview, IL: National Association of Neonatal Nurses.

National Association of Neonatal Nurse Practitioners. (2010b). *Standard for maintaining the competence of neonatal nurse practitioners* [Position Statement #3050]. Retrieved from http://www.nann.org/pdf /competence042910.pdf

National Association of Neonatal Nurses. (n.d.). *Neonatal developmental care specialist designation*. Retrieved from http://www.association-office.com /NANN/etools/products/testproducts.cfm?product_class=DCS

National Association of Neonatal Nurses. (2009a). *Educational preparation for nursing practice roles* [Position Statement #3048]. Retrieved from http://www.nann.org/pdf/09educational_prep.pdf

National Association of Neonatal Nurses. (2009b). *Educational standards and curriculum guidelines for neonatal nurse practitioner programs.* Retrieved from http://www.nann.org/pdf/09NNP_education_standards.pdf

National Association of Neonatal Nurses. (2010a). *NICU nurse involvement in ethical decisions* [Position Statement #3015, written in 1999, revised in 2006, reviewed in 2010]. Retrieved from http://www.nann.org/uploads /files/3015_reviewed_February_2010.pdf

National Association of Neonatal Nurses. (2010b). *Palliative care for newborns and infants* [Position Statement #3051]. Retrieved from http:// www.nann.org/uploads/files/Palliative_Care-final2-in_new _template_01-07-11.pdf

National Certification Corporation. (2011). *The National Certification Corporation certification exams.* Retrieved from http://www.nccwebsite .org/Certification

National Council of State Boards of Nursing. (2008). *Consensus model for APRN regulation: Licensure, accreditation, certification and education.* Retrieved from https://www.ncsbn.org/Consensus_Model_for_APRN _Regulation_July_2008.pdf

National Human Genome Project. (2010). *All about the Human Genome Project.* Retrieved from http://www.genome.gov/10001772#al-2

O'Grady, N. P., Alexander, M., Burns, L. A., Dellinger, E. P., Garland, J., Heard, S. O., . . . & Healthcare Infection Control Practices Advisory Committee (HICPAC). (2011). Guidelines for the prevention of intravascular catheter-related infections. *Clinical Infectious Diseases, 52*(4, Suppl.), S1–34.

Osterman, M. J. K., Martin, J. A., & Menacker, F. (2009, October 28). Expanded health data from the new birth certificate, 2006. *National Vital Statistics Reports, 58*(5). Hyattsville, MD: National Center for Health Statistics.

The presidency: The struggle of the baby boy. (1963, August 16). *Time.* Retrieved from http://www.time.com/time/subscriber/article /0,33009,894559-1,00.html

Price-Douglas, W., Romito, J., & Taylor, R. M. (2010). *Neonatal nursing transport standards: Guideline for practice* (3rd ed.). Glenview, IL: National Association of Neonatal Nurses.

Profit, J., Zupancic, J. A. F., Gould, J. B., & Petersen, L. A. (2007). Implementing pay-for-performance in the neonatal intensive care unit. *Pediatrics, 119*(5), 975–982.

Raju, T. N. K. (2011). From infant hatcheries to intensive care. In R. J. Martin, A. A. Fanaroff, & M. C. Walsh (Eds.). *Neonatal-perinatal medicine: Diseases of the fetus and infant*. St. Louis, MO: Elsevier.

Raju, T. N. K., Suresh, G., & Higgins, R. D. (2011). Patient safety in the context of neonatal intensive care: Research and educational opportunities. *Pediatric Research, 70*(1), 109–115.

Samra, H. A., McGrath, J. M., & Rollins, W. (2011). Patient safety in the NICU. *Journal of Perinatal & Neonatal Nursing, 25*(2), 123–132.

Siegel, R., Gardner, S. L., & Dickey, L. A. (2011). Families in crisis: Theoretical and practical considerations. In S. Gardner, B. Carter, M. Enzman-Hines, & J. Hernandez, (Eds.), *Neonatal intensive care* (7th ed., pp. 849–897). St. Louis, MO: Mosby Elsevier.

Stevens, K. R., & Harrison, L. (2007). Neonatal research and evidence-based practice. In C. Kenner & J. W. Lott (Eds.), *Comprehensive neonatal care: An interdisciplinary approach* (4th ed., pp. 594–605). St. Louis, MO: Saunders Elsevier.

Taylor, T., Massaro, A., Williams, L., Doering, J., McCarter, R., He, J., Talley, L., & Shoret, B. (2011). Effect of a dedicated percutaneously inserted central catheter team in neonatal catheter-related bloodstream infection. *Advances in Neonatal Care, 11*(2), 122–128.

Walden, M., & Gibbins, S. (2008). *Pain assessment and management: Guideline for practice* (2nd ed.). Glenview, IL: National Association of Neonatal Nurses.

Williams, P. H., & Sudia-Robinson, T. (2007). Legal and ethical issues of neonatal care. In C. Kenner & J. W. Lott (Eds.), *Comprehensive neonatal care: An interdisciplinary approach* (4th ed., pp. 606–614). St. Louis, MO: Saunders Elsevier.

World Health Organization. (2005). *The World Health Report 2005: Make every mother and child count.* Retrieved from http://www.who.int /whr/2005/en/index.html

World Health Organization. (2007). WHO launches "Nine patient safety solutions." Retrieved from http://www.who.int/mediacentre/news /releases/2007/pr22/en/index.html

World Health Organization. (2012). *Millennium Development Goal 4: Child mortality: Infant mortality.* Retrieved from http://apps.who.int /ghodata/?vid=240

Bibliography

American Academy of Pediatrics, Committee on the Fetus and Newborn. (2003). Advanced practice in neonatal nursing. *Pediatrics, 111*(6), 1453–1454.

Bracht, M., Kandankerv, A., Nodwell, S., & Stade, B. (2002). Cultural differences and parental responses to the preterm infant at risk: Strategies for supporting families. *Neonatal Network, 21*(6), 31–38.

Buffum, A. R., & Brandon, D. H. (2009). Mentoring new nurses in the neonatal intensive care unit: Impact on satisfaction and retention. *Journal of Perinatal & Neonatal Nursing, 23*(4), 357–362.

Cleveland, L. M. (2008). Parenting in the neonatal intensive care unit. *Journal of Obstetric, Gynecologic & Neonatal Nursing, 37*, 666–691.

deVonderweld, U., & Leonessa, M. (2009). Family centered neonatal care. *Early Human Development, 85*(10), 537–538.

Donn, S. M., & McDonnell, W. M. (2011). When bad things happen: Adverse event reporting and disclosure as patient safety and risk management tools in the neonatal intensive care unit. *American Journal of Perinatology.* Advance (online publication August 10, 2011) *29*(1), 65–70. (January.) Abstract retrieved from http://www.ncbi.nlm.nih.gov/pubmed/21833897.

International Council of Nurses. (2009). ICN of birth registration. Retrieved from http://www.icn.ch/images/stories/documents/publications/fact_sheets/10a_FS-Birth_Registration.pdf

Kenner, C., & Lott, J. W. (Eds.). (2007). *Comprehensive neonatal care: An interdisciplinary approach* (4th ed.). St. Louis, MO: Saunders Elsevier.

Kohn, K. T., Corrigan, J. M., & Donaldson, M. S. (Eds.). (2000). *To err is human: Building a safer health system.* Washington, DC: National Academy Press.

Lee, S. Y., & Weiss, S. J. (2009). When east meets west: Intensive care unit experiences among first-generation Chinese American parents. *Journal of Nursing Scholarship, 41*(3), 268–275.

Lefaiver, C. A., Lawlor-Klean, P., Welling, R., Smith, J., Waszak, L., & Micek, W. T. (2009). Using evidence to improve care for the vulnerable neonatal population. *Nursing Clinics of North America, 44*(1), 131–144.

McGrath, J. M. (2009). Mentoring nurses for the complexities of neonatal care. *Journal of Perinatal & Neonatal Nursing, 23*(2), 105–107.

Mundy, C. A. (2010). Assessment of family needs in neonatal intensive care units. *American Journal of Critical Care, 19*(2), 156–164.

Obeidat, H. M., Bond, E. A., & Callister, L. C. (2009). The parental experience of having an infant in the newborn intensive care unit. *Journal of Perinatal Education, 18*(3), 23–29.

Reis, M. D., Scott, S. D., & Rempel, G. R. (2009). Including parents in the evaluation of clinical microsystems in the neonatal intensive care unit. *Advances in Neonatal Care, 9*(4), 174–179.

Stokowski, L. A., Sansoucie, D. A., McDonald, K. O., Stein, J., Robinson, C., & Lovejoy, A. (2010). Advocacy: It is what we do. *Advances in Neonatal Care, 10*(2), 75–82.

Witt, C. (2007). Coping with ethical dilemmas in the NICU. *Advances in Neonatal Care, 7*(5), 217–218.

Appendix A.

Neonatal Nursing: Scope and Standards of Practice (2004)

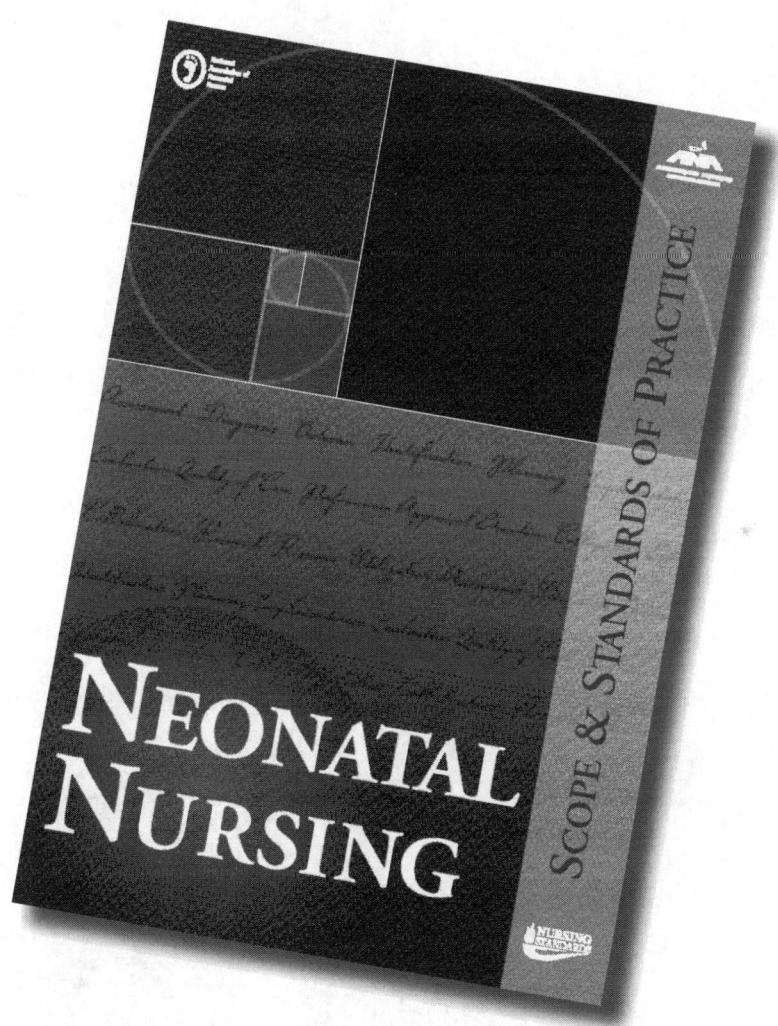

This appendix is not current and is of historical significance only.

This appendix is not current and is of historical significance only.

NEONATAL NURSING:
SCOPE AND STANDARDS
OF PRACTICE

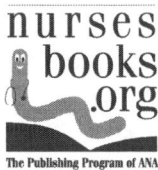

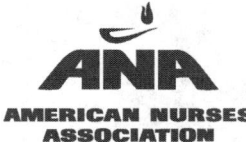

**AMERICAN NURSES
ASSOCIATION**

Washington, D.C.
2004

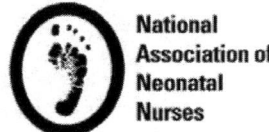

This appendix is not current and is of historical significance only.

Library of Congress Cataloging-in-Publication data

Neonatal nursing : scope and standards of practice.
    p. ; cm.
  Includes bibliographical references and index.
  ISBN 1-55810-222-1 (pbk.)
  ISBN 978-1-55810-222-4 (pbk.)
1. Infants (Newborn)—Diseases—Nursing—Standards.
  [DNLM: 1. Neonatal Nursing—standards. WY 157.3 N4388 2004]
  I. American Nurses Association. II. National Association of Neonatal Nurses.

  RJ253.N443 2004
  618.92'00231—dc22   2004011997

The American Nurses Association (ANA) is a national professional association. This ANA publication—*Neonatal Nursing: Scope and Standards of Practice*—reflects the thinking of the nursing profession on various issues and should be reviewed in conjunction with state board of nursing policies and practices. State law, rules, and regulations govern the practice of nursing, while *Neonatal Nursing: Scope and Standards of Practice* guides nurses in the application of their professional skills and responsibilities.

Published by nursesbooks.org
The Publishing Program of ANA

American Nurses Association
600 Maryland Avenue, SW • Suite 100 West • Washington, DC 20024
1-800-274-4ANA • http://www.nursingworld.org/

ISBN 1-55810-222-1
04SSVN   2M   05/04

This appendix is not current and is of historical significance only.

ACKNOWLEDGMENTS

This document was developed by the National Association of Neonatal Nurses (NANN) Scope and Standards Practice Task Force. The members of the task force gratefully acknowledge the work of the previous task forces that initiated the original documents on neonatal nursing practice. Carole Kenner, DNS RNC FAAN, especially is thanked for her review of the early drafts of this document.

The early versions of *Neonatal Nursing: Scope and Standards of Practice* were modified based on the thoughtful comments and editing suggestions of volunteer reviewers and from the pre-publication review by the NANN Board of Directors.

NANN Scope and Standards Task Force
Susan Stang, MSN, RNC, APN, Task Force Chair
Leda Afuang, MSN, RNC, LNC
Wendy Bedran, BSN, RN
Janet Geyer, MSN, RN, ARNP
Karen Goldschmidt, BSN, RNC
Cheryl King, MSN, CCRN

NANN Staff Liaisons
Brandon Dybala
Louise S. Miller, MA

NANN Board of Directors, 2003–2004
Catherine Witt, MS, RNC, NNP, President
Robin Bissinger, MSN, RNC, NNP, President-Elect
Peggy Gordin, MS, RNC, NNP, FAAN, Secretary
Suzanne Staebler, MSN, RNC, NNP, Treasurer
Margaret Conway-Orgel, MSN, RNC, NNP, Past President
Priscilla Frappier, MPH, MS, RNC, NNP, Director at Large
Karin Gracey, MSN, RNC, CNNP, Director at Large
Karen Kopischke, MS, RNC, NNP, Director at Large
Lori Sellers, MSN, RN, Director at Large
Cynthia Weiss, RNC, Director at Large
Linda Juretschke, MSN RNC NNP, Special Interest Group (SIG) Director at Large

American Nurses Association (ANA) Staff
Carol J. Bickford, PhD, RN,BC, Content Editor
Yvonne Humes, MSA
Winifred Carson-Smith, JD

This appendix is not current and is of historical significance only.

CONTENTS

This appendix is not current and is of historical significance only.

INTRODUCTION

Neonatal nursing, as a specialty, has developed significantly during the past 40 years. Specialty care for the sick or premature infant began with the invention of the incubator in 1878 and its subsequent display with infants at world expositions and fairs until the 1940s. In 1923 the first hospital center for premature infants in the United States was established, and in 1950 the first federal grant funding the Premature Institute program to train hospitals in caring for this special group of newborns was provided. These developments led to the expanded role of nurses into specialized nursing care for the neonate in the early 1960s and the country's first neonatal intensive care unit (NICU).

Advances in technology and health care led to regionalization in most large teaching hospitals and the development of high-tech neonatal care during the 1970s. The American College of Obstetricians and Gynecologists added validity to the specialty with the publication of standards of care for neonates. In turn, neonatal nurses developed their skills and advanced their roles in infant care as nurse clinicians, practitioners, clinical specialists, and educators.

As these well-trained nurses increased in number, they developed associations to further their knowledge and expertise. Developing from the Neonatal Nurses of Northern California, the Neonatal Nurses Association, and the Neonatal Nurse Clinicians Practitioners & Specialists, in 1984 the National Association of Neonatal Nurses (NANN) was born. Since its inception, NANN has provided the opportunity to specialize neonatal nursing further by consolidating the voice of its members and creating support and unity in this unique nursing field.

To help the profession and the public better understand the practice of neonatal nursing and thereby value today's neonatal nurses, the National Association of Neonatal Nurses convened the Scope and Standards of Practice Task Force to examine historical documents, references, and resources and then create the specialty's scope and standards of practice. This work identified key assumptions that guided further thinking and proved integral to the development of the scope of practice statement. (These assumptions are listed on page ix). The scope of practice statement provides the answers to the *who, what, where, when, why,* and *how* questions about the neonatal nursing specialty.

The standards for neonatal nursing practice are generic statements that define the responsibilities and accountability to the profession and the public of all registered nurses who care for high-risk neonates and their families.

This appendix is not current and is of historical significance only.

These standards reflect the values and priorities of the profession of nursing as they relate to the specialty of neonatal nursing and provide directives and a measurement framework for minimal levels of care that are common to the registered nurse in the neonatal nursing field.

The specialty scope and standards of practice must be considered in relation to the definition of nursing and other content in *Nursing's Social Policy Statement, 2nd Edition* (2003) and *Code of Ethics for Nurses with Interpretive Statements* (2001). As well, it must be reviewed and revised on a regular basis to reflect changes in health care and the nursing profession. In 2004, *Neonatal Nursing: Scope and Standards of Practice* completed the American Nurses Association's established review and recognition process for specialty nursing scope and standards of practice.

Considered together, *standards of practice* and *standards of professional performance* (ANA, 2004) encompass minimally acceptable levels of nursing care and nursing performance. The *standards of practice* include the steps in the nursing process: assessment, diagnosis, planning, implementation, and evaluation. In today's climate of cost containment and evidence-based practice, it must also include outcomes of care. The *standards of professional performance* include quality of care, performance appraisal, education, collegiality, ethics, collaboration, research, resource utilization, and leadership (ANA, 2004, p. 3). The professional nurse is expected to be competent and accountable in these areas of nursing practice.

This appendix is not current and is of historical significance only.

Underlying Assumptions

The following assumptions were made in the development of *Neonatal Nursing: Scope and Standards of Practice*:

1. The standards focus primarily on the process of providing nursing care to newborns/infants and their families.
2. The healthcare facility will provide a sufficient number of qualified registered nurses to deliver safe and effective neonatal nursing care.
3. Nursing care is individualized to meet the unique needs of each newborn/infant and family.
4. The nurse considers and respects the family's goals and preferences when developing and implementing a plan of care.
5. The nurse respects the cultural aspects of newborn/infant and family care.
6. The nurse respects the rights of the newborn/infant and family and manages information accordingly.
7. The nurse provides information to the family so informed decisions can be made regarding the care of the newborn/infant and family.
8. The nurse functions within the Nurse Practice Acts of the state and the established policies and procedures as described by the healthcare institution in which the nurse is practicing.
9. Nursing care is administered considering the rights of the patient and family, as outlined by the institution. Such care is given with regard for the family's spiritual and cultural values, in a manner that is ethically relevant, based on scientific knowledge, and within the confines of the legal system.
10. The nurse works in coordination with other healthcare providers to render care to the newborn/infant and family.
11. The nurse is expected to continue and maintain education within the neonatal specialty.
12. The nurse strives to provide a high quality of care while utilizing available resources.
13. The nurse promotes collegiality and collaboration in an effort to provide holistic care.
14. The nurse recognizes ethical dilemmas and use appropriate resources to work through these situations.
16. The nurse strives to ensure use of evidence-based care when possible and identify the need for research in areas lacking evidence to support practice.

This appendix is not current and is of historical significance only.

NEONATAL NURSING SCOPE OF PRACTICE

Neonatal nursing is the specialized care of the neonate, infant, and family from birth and hospitalization to discharge and follow-up care. Traditionally, this highly specialized nursing practice encompasses the care of infants born preterm, term, or ill from complications detected pre- or postnatally. Currently, the specialty has evolved to encompass care of the infant up to one year of age with problems that stem from complications of prematurity or other newborn illness. The neonatal nurse recognizes and respects each infant as a unique, individual human being, with the right to a pain-free, developmentally supportive care environment. The nurse assists the family's adaptation to a new, highly technical environment, while encouraging attachment to and bonding with their newborn. The neonatal nurse recognizes the family's attachment to the newborn as crucial for the infant's physical, psychological, and emotional wellbeing, growth, and development. The goal of the neonatal nurse is to empower the family through education, practice, and competence in caring for their newborn.

Practice Characteristics

Neonatal nurses understand complex newborn disease processes and acquire the expertise needed to utilize state-of-the-art technology to care for neonates and infants. The neonatal nurse has the ability to assess and manage care of the newborn infant and is able to respond appropriately to serious or life-threatening conditions. The neonatal nurse makes skilled, knowledgeable assessments of the infant, anticipates illness, and whenever possible prevents the occurrence of illness and injury or minimizes its effect. In caring for newborn infants, the neonatal nurse recognizes the importance of holistic care and supports the family's adaptive coping. Specific phenomena that form the framework for neonatal nursing practice include the following:

- *Communication:* Continual direct observation of the infant unable to communicate verbally is vital. The neonatal nurse detects subtle changes in the infant's physiological status and communicates these changes to the physician, advanced practice nurse, and family. The neonatal nurse works in collaboration with the healthcare team, including physicians, advanced practice nurses, case managers, laboratory technicians, occupational, physical, and respiratory therapists, nutritionists, social workers, and childlife specialists, to provide optimal care for the fragile newborn and family.

This appendix is not current and is of historical significance only.

- *Culturally Sensitive Care:* The neonatal nurse provides culturally sensitive care to the infant and family by understanding the family's unique cultural needs while caring for the newborn. Family-centered, culturally appropriate care can eliminate potential barriers to health care for the family and is essential for the infant's wellbeing (NANN, 1999b).

- *Developmental Care:* The neonatal nurse provides care for medically fragile infants while supporting their development, thereby enhancing the infant's growth and neurodevelopmental potential.

- *Health Promotion:* In planning and providing care, the neonatal nurse considers all aspects of the infant's health, including preventive health care. The neonatal nurse closely assesses the infant's physiological status, develops a specialized plan of care, and evaluates the infant's response. The neonatal nurse devises, coordinates, and executes an individualized plan of care for the newborn, revising plans as needed, and continually evaluates responses from the infant and family.

- *Environment:* The neonatal nurse recognizes the significant effects of the environment on the health of the newborn. The neonatal nurse identifies and treats pain and prevents suffering through management of the infant's discomfort with both independent nursing interventions and medications. The nurse strives to eliminate or minimize negative iatrogenic effects for the infant and to provide a nurturing environment; coordinates care to provide the infant with uninterrupted sleep periods; monitors the infant's temperature, comfort level, and nutritional needs; monitors the ambient lighting and noise level in the unit; and provides protection from infection. The neonatal nurse promotes positive family–infant interaction through holding, kangaroo care, breast or bottle feeding, and involvement in the infant's daily-care needs.

- *Discharge Planning:* The neonatal nurse plays an important role in preparing the family or caregivers for discharge of sick, medically fragile, or recovering term or preterm infants. The neonatal nurse must be knowledgeable of current, evidence-based discharge practices, and community resources to ease transition of infant and family into the home environment.

- *Ethical Decision-Making:* In practice, the neonatal nurse is challenged with ethical decisions daily. The nurse works in conjunction with physicians, advanced practice nurses, and family to provide care that is determined to be in the best interest of the child. The neonatal nurse acknowledges the parents' role as spokespersons for the infant. The neonatal nurse acts as infant advocate, providing the family with detailed information to enable fact-based decision-making and informed consent. The neonatal nurse identifies potential ethical conflicts and coordinates interdisciplinary forums for discussion and resolution.

This appendix is not current and is of historical significance only.

- *Family-Focused Care:* Neonatal nurses recognize the family as an integral part of the healthcare team, as well as the importance of the family's role in enhancing the developmental outcome of the infant. The neonatal nurse assists the family in caring for the newborn, whether that means teaching basic newborn care or teaching a family how to care for their medically fragile infant in the home. The nurse recognizes the infant's need of a family competent in physical care, as well as in interpreting behavioral cues.

- *Spiritual Care:* The neonatal nurse plays an integral role in helping families cope with hope and joy, as well as grief and loss. Extended hospitalization of the newborn is recognized as a family crisis. The neonatal nurse recognizes that grieving is individual and occurs in stages. The neonatal nurse learns and respects religious and spiritual family practices, while conveying acceptance, openness, and availability. The neonatal nurse assists the families and the infant at the end of life however possible.

- *Quality Assurance and Research:* The neonatal nurse utilizes research-based nursing practice to provide quality nursing care to the newborn. The nurse participates in identifying potential research studies to benefit the newborn and the practice of neonatal nursing care.

Practice Environment, Education, Certification, and Roles

The neonatal nurse provides health care to the infant in a variety of settings, including the delivery room, newborn nursery, and the subacute care, acute care, chronic care, transport, home care, and infant follow-up clinics. In the hospital setting, neonatal units are regionalized to provide care for specified infant-acuity levels. These units are typically described by the level of care they provide. The neonatal nurse has the opportunity to practice in environments with infants of varying degrees of acuity:

- *Delivery Room:* The neonatal nurse is responsible for attending the birth of every neonate deemed to be at high risk. Knowledge of common causes of infant distress at birth requiring neonatal resuscitation is essential. A nurse trained in neonatal resuscitation is responsible for rapid and accurate evaluation of the newborn at delivery.

- *Level I:* At this level of care, the nurse directly observes the neonate during the stabilization period after birth. The nurse monitors the infant's adaptation to extrauterine life and then ideally assists transition of the newborn to rooming in with the mother. The neonatal nurse can also practice in a newborn nursery taking care of healthy newborns. This level of care is an essential part of mother–infant care.

This appendix is not current and is of historical significance only.

- *Level II:* In the Level II setting, often referred to as special care or transitional care, the neonatal nurse takes on a greater responsibility for monitoring the premature newborn or the newborn who is having difficulty in adapting to extrauterine life. The neonatal nurse at this level cares for premature or term newborns who are ill or injured from complications at birth. The neonatal nurse provides the newborn with frequent observation and monitoring. The infants in this unit may require respiratory support, supplemental oxygen, intravenous therapy, specialized feeding, or time to mature prior to discharge. The nurse provides the family with discharge instruction and arranges for follow-up support when the infant is discharged to home.

- *Level III:* In the Level III unit (NICU), the neonatal nurse is challenged by treating the acutely ill newborn during a critical period. Expert care and knowledge are required in this highly technical and challenging environment. In the Level III neonatal unit, the nurse provides direct care for the premature or term infant who requires complex care. The neonatal nurse in this unit cares for the infant requiring intensive life-support techniques, such as mechanical ventilation, nitric oxide therapy, and high-frequency ventilation. Select Level III intensive care units have the added capability to care for an infant requiring extracorporeal membrane oxygenation (ECMO). The nurse in these units also cares for the chronically technology-dependent infant. The nurse teaches the family how to care for the child in the home setting or aids in the transition to a rehabilitation center (Bagwell et al., 2003).

- *Transport:* The neonatal nurse may be responsible for transporting an infant via ground or air. For those infants born acutely ill in a location without the necessary resources, the neonatal nurse assists the physician or advanced practice nurse in the transport to a tertiary care center (NANN, 1999c). The neonatal transport nurse is responsible for assessment, stabilization, and continuous high-level care during the transfer to the tertiary care center. The neonatal nurse may also be responsible for transporting the stable newborn back to the referring institution or a rehabilitation center.

The care of the neonatal patient is guided by the neonatal nursing standards of practice. At all care levels the neonatal nurse recognizes the importance of their role as an infant and family advocate. Training to assess minute changes in the infant's health and to observe unspoken cues and physiological changes define this nursing practice. The neonatal nurse evaluates outcomes of the infant's care and revises the plan as necessary to promote wellness. Sick newborns require the attention of specialized, expert neonatal nurses at all care levels.

This appendix is not current and is of historical significance only.

Graduation from an accredited nursing program and registered nursing licensure are required for entry into the field of neonatal nursing. An appropriate orientation program supports the registered nurse in initial practice. This program provides the nurse new to the field with the opportunity to work with an experienced neonatal nurse. The professional neonatal nurse is encouraged to meet their learning needs through professional development experiences, such as continuing education opportunities, conferences in neonatal care, and involvement in a professional nursing organization pertinent to practice.

Advanced practice neonatal nursing (APN) requires additional formal education at the master's degree level. The APN is an expert practitioner in the role of either nurse practitioner or clinical nurse specialist, who collaborates with neonatologists, pediatricians, and the infant's family (NANN, 1999a). The neonatal nurse practitioner (NNP) is a master's-prepared nurse who is responsible for managing a case load of infants, in collaboration with the neonatologist. The NNP typically is responsible for medical and nursing management of their patients, but also may be responsible for educating staff and developing standards of care. The neonatal clinical nurse specialist (NCNS), another master's-prepared neonatal nurse, is responsible for fostering continuous quality improvement in neonatal nursing care. The NCNS develops and educates staff, models expert nursing practice, and applies and promotes evidence-based nursing practice. Doctorate-prepared neonatal nurses may focus on conducting research to test caregiving practices and develop theory, while some are clinically focused. Both master's- and doctorate-prepared advanced practice neonatal nurses can teach neonatal nursing in the college or hospital setting (Harrigan et al., 2003).

Professionalism in neonatal nursing is demonstrated by assuming accountability for maintaining excellence in practice through self-motivated ventures as well as collaborative efforts with other nursing colleagues, organizations, and professional associations. Participation in the specialty's certification process further demonstrates the nurse's expertise in neonatal nursing. Nurses who have worked in neonatal nursing for a minimum of 2 years may choose to test their proficiency in neonatal nursing to become certified in either low-risk or high-risk neonatal nursing. Certification may be retained through continuing education or retesting.

Beyond the clinical environment and the provision of direct patient care, the neonatal nurse may practice in a variety of roles: clinical nurse specialist, educator, researcher, consultant, and clinical expert. Basic nursing roles include staff nurse, primary nurse, delivery room nurse, neonatal transport nurse, special care nurse, or transitional nursery nurse with varying degrees of advancement. Advanced-practice titles include clinical nurse specialist or nurse practitioner.

This appendix is not current and is of historical significance only.

Future Considerations

As technology advances, it may become possible to care for infants previously considered nonviable. The neonatal nurse's role will change as new technology and treatments are devised. Advances in infertility treatment continue to increase the need for neonatal nurses as the numbers of multiple births and high-risk deliveries increase.

Today, neonates are being discharged earlier than ever. There is a growing need for neonatal nurses to care for the newborn in the home. The nurse in this capacity will provide follow-up visits as well as technically advanced care for infants in the home. This trend requires well-developed care plans and communication between the NICU team and the home-care agency (Harrigan et al., 2003).

DNA testing and advances in gene therapy may have future implications for neonatal nurses. These advances may lead the way to preventing adverse genetic traits from being passed to future generations, thus preventing diseases such as Huntington's, Thalassaemia, Cystic Fibrosis, and Sickle Cell Disease. Another area of genetic research, Pharmacogenomics (combining genetics and pharmaceuticals), may enable medications to be adapted to an individual's genetic makeup, yielding more targeted drugs with fewer side effects, and replacing weight- and age-based dosing (Human Genome Project, 2004).

Fetal surgery has implications for this profession, merging the roles of the delivery room nurse, surgical nurse, and neonatal nurse. This type of surgery has the potential for creating new patient populations.

Ethical decision-making will continue to be an important part of the nurse's daily work, possibly becoming increasingly complex. It is important that neonatal nurses are nurtured and supported in this stressful environment. Recruitment and retention of neonatal nursing staff and support of new graduates entering the profession are crucial for the advancement and survival of the profession.

Through research, the neonatal nurse should strive to develop evidence-based practice guidelines. Much of the research in neonatology at present is physician-driven. The neonatal nurse has the opportunity to make changes in practice through scientifically grounded research studies. This will enable the neonatal nursing profession to grow and gain further professional credibility (Stevens, 2003).

This appendix is not current and is of historical significance only.

Due to all of the influences on preterm births, there will be a growing need for neonatal nurses in the future. There is a shortage of acute-care neonatal nurses, which is projected to continue into the next decade. Many health insurance plans are now providing reimbursement for the services of the APN and NNP in managing the low-risk and intermediate nursery in collaboration with physicians, because their services have proven to be advantageous and cost-effective.

This appendix is not current and is of historical significance only.

Standards of Neonatal Nursing Practice
Standards of Practice for Neonatal Nursing

Standard 1. Assessment

The neonatal nurse collects comprehensive data on the healthcare needs of the infant and family.

Measurement Criteria:

The neonatal nurse:

1. Determines the priority of data collection by the infant's and family's immediate condition and needs.

2. Collects data including antenatal and perinatal information, pertinent sociocultural data, physical assessment data, laboratory data analyses, and diagnostic testing.

3. Collects pertinent data using appropriate assessment techniques.

4. Utilizes data sources including family members, significant others, and other healthcare providers. Reassessment should be completed within a reasonable time, to ensure that the needs of the infant and family continue to be met.

5. Employs a data collection process that is systematic, ongoing, and relevant to the changing healthcare needs of the infant and the learning needs of the family.

6. Collects relevant data, systematically documented in a retrievable form.

7. Analyzes data to produce information about the infant's needs for treatment and services, to identify the need for additional data, and to identify patterns and variances.

8. Collects relevant data regarding the continued needs of the infant and family during follow-up visits and convalescent periods.

9. Assesses the infant for the presence of pain, then treats and reassesses in accordance with the institution's process.

Additional Measurement Criteria for the Advanced Practice Registered Nurse:

The advanced practice registered nurse initiates and interprets diagnostic tests and procedures relevant to the infant's current status.

This appendix is not current and is of historical significance only.

STANDARD 2. DIAGNOSIS

The neonatal nurse formulates diagnoses based on analysis and synthesis of assessment data.

Measurement Criteria:

The neonatal nurse:

1.   Derives diagnoses using assessment data that reflect the infant's current clinical condition.

2.   Refines and revises diagnoses regularly, based on data subsequently collected.

3.   Validates diagnoses with the infant's family and other healthcare providers when possible.

4.   Derives diagnoses encompassing:

   •   the infant's identified or potential physiological and developmental problems,

   •   the infant's integration into the family during the period of hospitalization and after discharge,

   •   the support and educational needs of the family, and

   •   any present or potential environmental problems.

5.   Documents diagnoses in a manner that facilitates the determination of expected outcomes and the plan of care.

Additional Measurement Criteria for the Advanced Practice Registered Nurse:

The advanced practice registered nurse:

•   Systematically compares and contrasts clinical findings with normal and abnormal variations and developmental events in formulating a differential diagnosis.

•   Utilizes complex data and information obtained during review of history, interview, examination, and diagnostic procedures in identifying diagnoses.

•   Assists staff in developing and maintaining competency in the diagnostic process.

This appendix is not current and is of historical significance only.

STANDARD 3. OUTCOME IDENTIFICATION

The neonatal nurse identifies expected individualized outcomes of care based on the needs of the infant and family.

Measurement Criteria:

The neonatal nurse:

1. Derives outcomes from the assessment and relevant nursing diagnoses.

2. Identifies outcomes consistent with current scientific evidence.

3. Mutually formulates outcomes with input from other healthcare providers and the family whenever possible.

4. Ensures that outcomes are culturally appropriate and realistic in relation to the infant and the family's present and potential capabilities.

5. Derives outcomes that are attainable in relation to the resources available to the infant and the family.

6. Develops a realistic time frame for attainment of objectives.

7. Identifies outcomes that provide direction for continuity of care.

8. Derives outcomes that provide a basis for evaluating and monitoring care.

Additional Measurement Criteria for the Advanced Practice Registered Nurse:

The advanced practice registered nurse:

• Identifies expected outcomes that incorporate scientific evidence and are achievable through implementation of evidence-based practices.

• Identifies expected outcomes that incorporate cost and clinical effectiveness, family or caregiver satisfaction, and continuity and consistency among providers.

• Supports the use of clinical guidelines linked to positive infant outcomes.

This appendix is not current and is of historical significance only.

STANDARD 4. PLANNING

The neonatal nurse develops a plan of care that prescribes interventions to attain expected outcomes.

Measurement Criteria:

The neonatal nurse:

1. Develops a plan that is individualized to the infant and family and is culturally, environmentally, and educationally sensitive and age-appropriate.

2. Develops the plan with the family and other healthcare providers whenever appropriate.

3. Ensures that the plan reflects current neonatal nursing practice.

4. Organizes, integrates, and plans care with consideration for the infant's stage of development.

5. Develops a plan that incorporates the family in caregiving based on the infant's condition and the family's ability to participate.

6. Ensures that the plan is systematically documented and easily retrievable.

7. Provides for continuity of care within the plan.

8. Ensures that the plan is a dynamic process that addresses the needs of the infant. It must be reevaluated within a reasonable time to ensure that the needs of the infant continue to be met.

9. Establishes the plan priorities for care with the family and other healthcare providers.

10. Integrates into the plan current trends and research affecting care in the planning process.

Additional Measurement Criteria for the Advanced Practice Registered Nurse:

The advanced practice registered nurse:

*   Identifies assessment, diagnostic strategies, and therapeutic interventions within the plan that reflect current evidence, including data, research, literature, and expert clinical knowledge.

*   Selects or designs strategies to meet the multifaceted needs of special-care infants and their families or caregivers.

*   Includes the synthesis of family or caregiver values and beliefs regarding nursing and medical therapies within the plan.

This appendix is not current and is of historical significance only.

STANDARD 5. IMPLEMENTATION

The neonatal nurse implements the plan of care.

Measurement Criteria:

The neonatal nurse:

1. Ensures that implementation of care is systematic and ongoing.

2. Utilizes interventions that are consistent with the established plan of care.

3. Organizes interventions to provide an environment that supports the infant's physical and developmental wellbeing.

4. Implements interventions in a manner that promotes family involvement and acquisition of progressive caregiving skills.

5. Implements interventions in a safe, timely, and appropriate manner.

6. Documents interventions in a retrievable form.

7. Individualizes interventions based on the specific needs of the infant and family.

Additional Measurement Criteria for the Advanced Practice Registered Nurse:

The advanced practice registered nurse:

*   Facilitates utilization of systems and community resources to implement the plan.

*   Supports collaboration with nursing colleagues and other disciplines to implement the plan.

*   Incorporates new knowledge and strategies to initiate change in nursing care practices if desired outcomes are not achieved.

This appendix is not current and is of historical significance only.

STANDARD 5A: COORDINATION OF CARE

The neonatal nurse coordinates care delivery.

Measurement Criteria:

The neonatal nurse:

1. Coordinates implementation of the plan.

2. Documents the coordination of the care.

Additional Measurement Criteria for the Advanced Practice Registered Nurse:

The advanced practice registered nurse:

- Provides leadership in the coordination of multidisciplinary health care for integrated delivery of infant care services.

- Synthesizes data and information to prescribe necessary system and community support measures, including environmental modifications.

- Coordinates system and community resources that enhance delivery of care across continuums.

This appendix is not current and is of historical significance only.

STANDARD 5B: HEALTH TEACHING AND HEALTH PROMOTION

The neonatal nurse employs strategies to promote health and a safe environment.

Measurement Criteria:

The neonatal nurse:

1. Provides family or caregiver teaching that addresses such topics as healthy lifestyles, risk-reducing behaviors, developmental needs, and normal/specific infant care and safety.

2. Uses health promotion and health teaching methods appropriate to the situation and the family or caregiver's developmental level, learning needs, readiness, ability to learn, language preference, and culture.

3. Seeks opportunities for feedback and evaluation of the effectiveness of the strategies used.

Additional Measurement Criteria for the Advanced Practice Registered Nurse:

The advanced practice registered nurse:

• Synthesizes empirical evidence on risk behaviors, learning theories, behavioral change theories, motivational theories, epidemiology, and other related theories and frameworks when designing health information and family or caregiver education.

• Designs health information and family or caregiver education appropriate to the family or caregiver's developmental level, learning needs, readiness to learn, and cultural values and beliefs.

• Evaluates health information resources, such as the Internet, within the area of practice for accuracy, readability, and comprehensibility to help the family or caregiver access quality health information.

This appendix is not current and is of historical significance only.

STANDARD 5C: CONSULTATION

The advanced practice registered nurse provides consultation to influence the identified plan, enhance the abilities of others, and effect change.

Additional Measurement Criteria for the Advanced Practice Registered Nurse:

The advanced practice registered nurse:

- Synthesizes clinical data, theoretical frameworks, and evidence when providing consultation.

- Facilitates the effectiveness of a consultation by involving the family or caregiver in decision-making and negotiating role responsibilities.

- Communicates consultation recommendations that facilitate change.

STANDARD 5D: PRESCRIPTIVE AUTHORITY AND TREATMENT

The advanced practice registered nurse uses prescriptive authority, procedures, referrals, treatments, and therapies in accordance with state and federal laws and regulations.

Additional Measurement Criteria for the Advanced Practice Registered Nurse:

The advanced practice registered nurse:

- Prescribes evidence-based treatments, therapies, and procedures considering the infant's comprehensive healthcare needs.

- Prescribes pharmacologic agents based on a current knowledge of pharmacology and physiology.

- Prescribes specific pharmacological agents or treatments based on clinical indicators, the infant's status and needs, and the results of diagnostic and laboratory tests.

- Evaluates therapeutic and potential adverse effects of pharmacological and non-pharmacological treatments.

- Provides the family or caregiver with information about intended effects and potential adverse effects of proposed prescriptive therapies.

- Provides information about costs, alternative treatments, and procedures, as appropriate.

This appendix is not current and is of historical significance only.

STANDARD 6. EVALUATION

The neonatal nurse evaluates the progress of the infant and family toward the attainment of established, expected outcomes.

Measurement Criteria:

The neonatal nurse:

1. Evaluates care in a systematic, ongoing, and criterion-based manner.

2. Evaluates interventions in relation to desired, expected outcomes, and alters them when warranted.

3. Evaluates interventions based on the infant's physiological and behavioral responses, and alters them when warranted.

4. Uses ongoing assessment data to revise diagnoses, outcomes, and the plan of care as needed.

5. Systematically documents revisions in the infant's plan of care and reports to appropriate members of the healthcare team.

6. Involves the infant's family or caregivers and other healthcare providers in the evaluation process when appropriate.

7. Documents the infant's and family or caregiver's responses to interventions in a retrievable form.

Additional Measurement Criteria for the Advanced Practice Registered Nurse:

The advanced practice registered nurse:

- Evaluates the accuracy of the diagnosis and effectiveness of the interventions in relationship to the infant's and the family's or caregiver's attainment of expected outcomes.

- Synthesizes the results of the evaluation analyses to determine the impact of the plan on the affected infants, families, groups, communities, and institutions.

- Uses the results of the evaluation analyses to make or recommend process or structural changes including policy, procedure or protocol documentation, as appropriate.

This appendix is not current and is of historical significance only.

STANDARDS OF PROFESSIONAL PERFORMANCE FOR NEONATAL NURSING

STANDARD 7. QUALITY OF PRACTICE

The neonatal nurse systematically evaluates the quality and effectiveness of nursing practice.

Measurement Criteria:

The neonatal nurse:

1. Participates in activities to assess the quality of care that are appropriate to the nurse's education and position. These activities may include the following:

    • Identification of aspects of care that affect quality.

    • Analysis of quality data to identify opportunities for improvement of care.

    • Development of policies, procedures, and practice guidelines reflective of quality of care.

    • Identification of indicators used to monitor quality and affect neonatal care.

    • Ongoing data collection for monitoring the quality and effectiveness of nursing care.

    • Articulation of recommendations for quality improvement of nursing practice or patient outcomes.

    • Participation in interdisciplinary teams to implement activities and evaluate clinical practice or health issues.

2. Uses continuous quality-improvement activities to initiate changes in nursing practice.

3. Uses quality-improvement data to initiate healthcare delivery system changes, as needed.

4. Works in collaboration with the healthcare team to use scientific research to provide evidence-based practice.

This appendix is not current and is of historical significance only.

Additional Measurement Criteria for the Advanced Practice Registered Nurse:

The advanced practice registered nurse:

- Obtains and maintains professional certification in neonatal nursing.
- Designs quality improvement initiatives.
- Implements initiatives to evaluate the need for change.
- Evaluates the practice environment and quality of nursing care rendered in relation to existing evidence, identifying opportunities for research.

STANDARD 8. EDUCATION

The neonatal nurse acquires and maintains current knowledge and competency in nursing practice.

Measurement Criteria:

The neonatal nurse:

1. Participates in ongoing educational activities related to clinical and theoretical knowledge and professional issues.
2. Seeks experiences that reflect current clinical practice to maintain current clinical skills and competence.
3. Acquires knowledge and skills appropriate to the neonatal specialty and practice setting.

Additional Measurement Criteria for the Advanced Practice Registered Nurse:

The advanced practice registered nurse uses current healthcare research findings and other evidence to expand clinical knowledge, enhance role performance, and increase knowledge of professional issues.

This appendix is not current and is of historical significance only.

STANDARD 9. PROFESSIONAL PRACTICE EVALUATION

The neonatal nurse evaluates one's own nursing practice in relation to professional practice standards and guidelines, relevant statutes, rules, and regulations.

Measurement Criteria:

The neonatal nurse's practice conforms with current practice standards, guidelines, statutes, rules, and regulations.

The neonatal nurse:

1.   Engages in performance appraisal on a regular basis, identifying areas of strengths as well as areas for professional development.

2.   Seeks constructive feedback on an ongoing basis for the purpose of professional development.

3.   Takes action to achieve professional goals identified during the performance appraisal process.

4.   Participates in peer review as appropriate.

5.   Demonstrates knowledge of current professional practice standards, laws, and regulations in their own individual practice.

Additional Measurement Criteria for the Advanced Practice Registered Nurse:

The advanced practice registered nurse engages in a formal process seeking feedback regarding one's own practice from peers, professional colleagues, and others.

This appendix is not current and is of historical significance only.

STANDARD 10. COLLEGIALITY

The neonatal nurse interacts with, and contributes to the professional development of, peers, other healthcare providers, and team members as colleagues.

Measurement Criteria:

The neonatal nurse:

1. Shares knowledge and skills with colleagues.

2. Provides peers with constructive feedback regarding neonatal care and practice.

3. Interacts with colleagues to enhance one's own professional neonatal nursing practice.

4. Contributes to an environment that is conducive to the clinical education of nursing students, other healthcare trainees, and other employees, as appropriate.

5. Contributes to a supportive and healthy work environment.

Additional Measurement Criteria for the Advanced Practice Registered Nurse:

The advanced practice registered nurse:

•   Models expert practice to interdisciplinary team members and healthcare consumers.

•   Mentors other nurses and colleagues as appropriate.

•   Participates with interdisciplinary teams that contribute to role development and advanced nursing practice and health care.

This appendix is not current and is of historical significance only.

STANDARD 11. COLLABORATION

The neonatal nurse collaborates with the family or caregiver and others in the conduct of nursing practice.

Measurement Criteria:

The neonatal nurse:

1. Communicates with the family and other healthcare providers regarding neonatal care and nursing's role in the provision of care.

2. Collaborates with the family and other healthcare providers in the formulation of overall goals and the plan of care, and in healthcare decisions related to the care and the delivery of services.

3. Consults with other healthcare providers for neonatal care, as needed.

4. Initiates referrals, including provisions for continuity of care, as needed.

Additional Measurement Criteria for the Advanced Practice Registered Nurse:

The advanced practice registered nurse:

•   Partners with other disciplines to enhance infant care through interdisciplinary activities such as education, consultation, management, technological development, or research opportunities.

•   Facilitates an interdisciplinary process with other members of the healthcare team.

•   Documents plan of care communications, rationales for plan of care changes, and collaborative discussions to improve infant care.

This appendix is not current and is of historical significance only.

STANDARD 12. ETHICS

The neonatal nurse's decisions and actions on behalf of infants and their families or caregivers in all areas of practice are determined in an ethical manner.

Measurement Criteria:

The neonatal nurse:

1. Ensures that their practice is guided by *Nursing's Social Policy Statement, 2nd Edition* (ANA 2003) and *Code of Ethics for Nurses with Interpretive Statements* (ANA, 2001).

2. Maintains patient and family confidentiality within legal and regulatory parameters.

3. Acts as a patient advocate and assists the family in developing skills to become advocates for their child.

4. Delivers care in a nonjudgmental and nondiscriminatory manner that is sensitive to patient diversity.

5. Delivers care in a manner that preserves patient and family autonomy, dignity, and rights from first encounter through end-of-life care.

6. Utilizes available resources in formulating ethical decisions.

Additional Measurement Criteria for the Advanced Practice Registered Nurse:

The advanced practice registered nurse:

•   Informs the family, caregiver, or other decision-maker of the risks, benefits, and outcomes of healthcare regimens.

•   Participates in multidisciplinary teams that evaluate ethical risks, benefits, and outcomes.

This appendix is not current and is of historical significance only.

STANDARD 13. RESEARCH

The neonatal nurse integrates research findings into practice.

Measurement Criteria:

The neonatal nurse:

1. Utilizes the best available evidence (ideally scientific research findings) to develop the plan of care and interventions and guide practice decisions.

2. Participates in research activities at various levels appropriate to the nurse's education, experience, and position. These may include the following:

   • Identification of clinical problems pertinent to neonatal nursing care.

   • Participation in all aspects of the research process, as appropriate, including data collection.

   • Participation in unit, organizational, community, or global research activities.

   • Dissemination of research information and findings with peers and others.

   • Conducting research.

   • Critiquing of research for application to neonatal practice.

   • Use of research findings in the development of policies, procedures, and practice guidelines for neonatal care.

   • Use of research findings to advance the state of nursing science in the care of neonatal patients and families.

Additional Measurement Criteria for the Advanced Practice Registered Nurse:

The advanced practice registered nurse:

• Contributes to nursing knowledge by conducting or synthesizing research that discovers, examines and evaluates knowledge, theories, criteria, and creative approaches to improve healthcare practice.

• Formally disseminates research findings through activities such as presentations, publications, consultation, and journal clubs.

This appendix is not current and is of historical significance only.

STANDARD 14. RESOURCE UTILIZATION

The neonatal nurse considers factors related to safety, effectiveness, cost, and impact on practice in the planning and delivering of nursing services.

Measurement Criteria:

The neonatal nurse:

1. Evaluates factors such as patient safety, effectiveness, availability, and cost when choosing among practice options having the same expected patient outcome.

2. Assists the family in identifying and securing necessary resources and services to address healthcare needs.

3. Assigns or delegates tasks as defined by the state Nurse Practice Acts and in accordance with the designated caregiver's knowledge, experience, and skills.

4. Assigns or delegates tasks based on the needs and condition of the infant, the potential for harm, the stability of the infant's condition, the complexity of the care, and the predictability of the outcome.

5. Assists the family or caregivers in becoming informed consumers with regard to risks, benefits, and cost of treatment and care.

Additional Measurement Criteria for the Advanced Practice Registered Nurse:

The advanced practice registered nurse:

- Utilizes organizational and community resources to formulate a multidisciplinary plan of care.

- Develops innovative solutions for infant care problems that address effective resource utilization and maintenance of quality.

- Develops evaluation strategies to demonstrate cost effectiveness, cost benefit, and efficiency factors associated with neonatal nursing practice.

This appendix is not current and is of historical significance only.

STANDARD 15. LEADERSHIP

The neonatal nurse provides leadership in the professional practice setting and the profession.

Measurement Criteria:

The neonatal nurse:

1. Engages in teamwork as a team player and a team builder.

2. Works to create and maintain healthy environments in local, regional, national, or international communities.

3. Displays the ability to define a clear vision, the associated goals, and a plan to implement and measure progress.

4. Demonstrates a commitment to continuous, lifelong learning for self and others.

5. Teaches others to succeed by mentoring and other strategies.

6. Exhibits creativity and flexibility through times of change.

7. Demonstrates energy, excitement, and a passion for quality work.

8. Willingly accepts mistakes by self and others, thereby creating a culture in which risk-taking is not only accepted, but expected.

9. Inspires loyalty through valuing of people as the most precious asset in an organization.

10. Directs the coordination of care across settings and among caregivers, including supervision of licensed and unlicensed personnel in any assigned or delegated tasks.

11. Serves in key roles in the work setting by participating on committees, councils, and administrative teams.

12. Promotes advancement of the profession through participation in professional organizations.

This appendix is not current and is of historical significance only.

Additional Measurement Criteria for the Advanced Practice Registered Nurse:

The advanced practice registered nurse:

- Works to influence policymaking bodies to improve infant care.

- Provides direction to enhance the effectiveness of the healthcare team.

- Initiates and revises protocols or guidelines to reflect evidence-based practice, to reflect accepted changes in care management, or to address emerging problems.

- Promotes communication and the advancement of the profession through writing, publishing, and presentations for professional or lay audiences.

- Designs innovations to effect change in practice and to improve health outcomes.

This appendix is not current and is of historical significance only.

GLOSSARY

Assessment. A systematic data collection process used by the nurse, through interaction with the infant and family, significant others, and healthcare providers, to collect and analyze information regarding the health needs of the infant and family. Information collected may be related to the physiological, psychosocial, sociocultural, spiritual, environmental, educational, developmental, and discharge-planning needs of the infant and family. These data can be collected through observation, physical examination, medical record review, interviews, and discussion with family members, as well as perinatal, neonatal, and other healthcare providers, as appropriate.

Collaboration. Planning, implementing, and evaluating care, with consideration given to each discipline and the family's unique contribution to the care. Similar to collegiality, in that both require teamwork to achieve the desired care outcome.

Collegiality. A work ethic that involves working as a team in a professional and equal manner to achieve the expected care outcome.

Diagnosis. A clinical judgment made by a nurse regarding the infant or family responses to actual or potential health conditions or needs. Diagnoses provide the basis for determining a plan of care that will achieve expected outcomes.

Education. The degree to which the nurse keeps academically current in the neonatal nursing specialty.

Environment. The conditions, circumstances, and influences surrounding and affecting the infant and family, including the physical and caregiving environments. The physical environment refers to conditions such as lighting and noise levels and temperature fluctuations within an ambient space. The caregiving environment refers to the manner in which interventions are administered, the way the infant and family are handled, and the use of equipment when administering care (Gottfried, 1985).

Evaluation. The determination of the infant and family's progress toward the attainment of expected outcomes and the effectiveness of the nursing care delivered by the professional nurse; the final step in the nursing process.

Expected outcomes. Goals achieved as a result of care that can be objectively measured.

This appendix is not current and is of historical significance only.

Family. Family of origin, significant others, or caregivers.

Guidelines. Recommended courses of action in various clinical situations or for specific client conditions or populations. Guidelines provide linkages among nursing diagnoses, interventions, and outcome. They also describe alternatives available to each patient and provide a basis for the evaluation of care and allocation of resources. Guidelines are recommendations for practice with supportive evidence from the literature.

Implementation. Activities used by the nurse to carry out the plan of care, including psychomotor skills, interviews, and coordination and delegation of care activities.

Infant. A baby in the first year of life.

Kangaroo care. The practice of resting an infant on a parent's bare chest to promote parent–infant bonding in babies requiring special care. Other benefits include earlier discharge from hospital, easier breast-feeding, and mutual comfort.

Neonate, Newborn. An infant 28 days of age or younger.

Performance appraisal. Measurement of the cognitive and behavioral aspects of the neonatal nurse's role.

Performance standards. Broad statements of professional nursing expectations. They include competencies and accountabilities for the professional nurse. They reflect criteria that are measurable.

Planning. Documenting the care to be delivered to the infant and family to attain the expected outcomes.

Quality of care. The degree to which the care rendered reflects the expected minimum level of care and the achievement of expected care outcomes, according to defined professional and consumer expectations.

Research. The systematic study of care practices or professional performance. Research yields evidence to support interventions.

Resource utilization. Awareness of the supports available and necessary for care, as well as use of those supports in a responsible manner to achieve quality of care.

Standards. Broad statements that address the basic scope of professional nursing practice. They identify minimum acceptable care practices for the professional nurse who cares for specific populations of patients. These standards are population-based and not setting-specific.

This appendix is not current and is of historical significance only.

REFERENCES

American Nurses Association. (2001). *Code of ethics for nurses with interpretive statements*. Washington, DC: American Nurses Publishing. (See also http://www.nursingworld.org/ethics/ecode.htm)

American Nurses Association. (2003). *Nursing's social policy statement, 2nd edition*. Washington, DC: nursesbooks.org.

American Nurses Association (2004). *Nursing: Scope and standards of practice*. Washington, DC: nursesbooks.org.

Bagwell et al. (2003) Regionalization in today's healthcare delivery system. In Kenner, C. & Wright Lott, J., editors, *Comprehensive neonatal nursing, 3rd Edition*. St. Louis, MO: Mosby.

Harrigan, R.C. & Perez, D.J. (2003). Neonatal nursing in the new healthcare delivery environment. In Kenner, C. & Wright Lott, J., editors. *Comprehensive neonatal nursing, 3rd Edition*. St. Louis, MO: Mosby.

Human Genome Project. (2004). www.ornl.gov/sci/technsource/Human_Genome/home.shtml

Joint Commission on Accreditation of Healthcare Organizations. (2003). *Comprehensive accreditation manual for hospitals*. Oakbrook Terrace, IL: JCAHO.

National Association of Neonatal Nurses. (1999a). *Advanced practice neonatal nurse role* (No. 3000). Glenview, IL: NANN.

National Association of Neonatal Nurses. (1999b). *Cultural competence* (No. 3037). Glenview, IL: NANN.

National Association of Neonatal Nurses. (1999c). *Transport of neonates across state lines* (No. 3020). Glenview, IL: NANN.

Stevens, K.R. (2003). Evidence-based neonatal nursing practice. In Kenner, C. & Wright Lott, J., editors. *Comprehensive neonatal nursing, 3rd Edition*. St. Louis, MO: Mosby.

(*Note*: All URLs were confirmed active as of March 30, 2004.)

This appendix is not current and is of historical significance only.

BIBLIOGRAPHY

American Academy of Pediatrics. (2000). *Policy statement prevention and management of pain stress in the neonate* (RE9945). Elk Grove Village, IL: AAP.

American Academy of Pediatrics and American College of Obstetricians and Gynecologists. (2002). *Guidelines for perinatal care, 5th Ed.* Elk Grove Village, IL: AAP.

American Nurses Association. (2001). Press release: ANA House of Delegates Passes Revised Code of Ethics. Washington, DC: ANA.

American Nurses Association (2002). *Scope and standards of neuroscience nursing practice.* Washington, DC: American Nurses Publishing.

Association of Women's Health, Obstetric, and Neonatal Nurses. (1997). *Guidelines of neonatal nursing: Orientation and development for Registered and Advanced Practice Nurses in basic and intensive care settings.* Washington, DC: AWHONN.

Association of Women's Health, Obstetric, and Neonatal Nurses. (1998). *Standards and guidelines for professional nursing practice in the care of women and newborns, 5th Ed.* Washington, DC: AWHONN.

Carrera, J.M., Chervenak, F.A., and Kurjak, A. (2003). *Controversies in perinatal medicine: The fetus as a patient.* Boca Raton, FL: CRC Press-Parthenon Publishers. (This book was developed from the 2003 proceedings in Barcelona, Spain, of the 19th International Congress of the Society of the Fetus as Patient.)

Carter, B.S. (2001). *Ethical issues in neonatal care.* www.emedicine.com

Gottfried, A.W. (1985). Environment of newborn in special care units. In Gottfried, A.W. & Gaiter, J.L. eds. *Infant stress under intensive care.* Baltimor University Park Press.

National Association of Neonatal Nurses. (1999). *NICU nurse involvement in ethical decisions (Treatment of critically ill newborns).* (No. 3015). Glenview, IL: NANN.

National Association of Neonatal Nurses. (1999). *Standards of care for neonatal nursing practice.* Glenview, IL: NANN.

National Association of Neonatal Nurses. (2003). *FAQs.* www.nann.org

National Association of Neonatal Nurses. (2003). *History.* www.nann.org

This appendix is not current and is of historical significance only.

Brophy, M.S.S. (2001). Nurse advocacy in the neonatal unit: Putting theory into practice. *Journal of Neonatal Nursing,* 7(1) 10–11.

Smington, A. & Pinelli, J. (2003). *Developmental care for promoting development and preventing morbidity in preterm infants.* Cochrane Library *(Cochrane Review).*

World Health Organization. (2004). *Child and adolescent health and development: Prevention and care of Illness: Neonates and infants.* Geneva: WHO. http://www.who.int/child-adolescent-health/

(*Note:* All URLs were confirmed active as of March 30, 2004.)

Index

Note: Entries with [2004] indicate an entry from *Neonatal Nursing: Scope and Standards of Practice* (2004), reproduced in Appendix A. That information is not current but included for historical value only.

A

AACN. *See* American Association of Critical-Care Nurses (AACN)

AAP. *See* American Academy of Pediatrics (AAP)

Abilities in neonatal nursing practice, 11, 30
  See also Knowledge, skills, abilities, and judgment

Accountability in neonatal nursing practice, 16
  leadership and, 44
  quality of practice and, 41

Advanced practice registered nurses (APRNs) in neonatal nursing practice, 16
  assessment competencies, 20
    measurement criteria [2004], 78
  collaboration competencies, 46–47
    measurement criteria [2004], 91

collegiality, measurement criteria [2004], 90

consultation competencies, 32
  measurement criteria [2004], 85

coordination of care
  competencies, 29
  measurement criteria [2004], 83

diagnosis competencies, 22
  measurement criteria [2004], 79

education competencies, 38
  measurement criteria [2004], 88

environmental health competencies, 51–52

ethics competencies, 37
  measurement criteria [2004], 92

evaluation competencies, 34–35
  measurement criteria [2004], 86

evidence-based practice and research competencies, 40

health teaching and promotion
  competencies, 30–31
  measurement criteria [2004], 84

M

Maternal health, 6

Medical errors, 12, 46

Midwives, 3

Mother–baby unit, 13

N

NANNP. *See* National Association
of Neonatal Nurse Practitioners
(NANNP)

NANN. *See* National Association of
Neonatal Nurses (NANN)

National Association of Neonatal Nurse
Practitioners (NANNP), 16

National Association of Neonatal Nurses
(NANN), viii

National Certification Corporation
(NCC), 16

National Council of State Boards of
Nursing (NCSBN), 17

NCC. *See* National Certification
Corporation (NCC)

NCNS. *See* Neonatal clinical nurse
specialist (NCNS)

NCSBN. *See* National Council of State
Boards of Nursing (NCSBN)

Neonatal clinical nurse specialist
(NCNS), 17

Neonatal intensive care unit (NICU), 2,
4, 6, 11, 12, 14, 18

Neonatal nursing practice
See also Scope of neonatal nursing
practice; Neonatal registered
nurses
defined, 53
levels of care and, 13–15

Neonatal nurse practitioners (NNPs), 17
advocacy, 11
assumptions, 4–5
certification, 16–17
characteristics, 5–6
continuous assessment, 6–7
culturally sensitive care, 9
definition, 1–3
discharge planning, 10–11
education, 16–17
environment, 8
ethical decision-making, 10
evidence-based practice, 11–12
family-focused care, 8
future considerations, 17–18
health promotion, 7
history, 3–4
levels of care, 13–15
overview, 1–3
patient safety, 12
quality assurance, 11–12
research, 12–13
roles in, 16–17
spiritual care, 9
[2004], 68–98
See also Neonatal registered nurses

Neonatal registered nurses, 7, 8, 9, 10, 16
assessment competencies, 19–20
measurement criteria [2004], 78
collaboration competencies, 46–47
measurement criteria [2004], 91
collegiality measurement criteria
[2004], 90
communication competencies, 43
coordination of care competencies, 29
measurement criteria [2004], 83
diagnosis competencies, 21
measurement criteria [2004], 79
education competencies, 38
measurement criteria [2004], 88
environmental health competencies, 51

See also Cultural competence and sensitivity

ventilators, 3, 4

Vermont Oxford Network (quality and safety of care), 12

Vigilance, neonatal nursing practice, 6–7

W

Work and practice environments for neonatal nursing practice, 6, 7, 8, 12, 17

collaboration and, 46

competencies involving, 19, 28, 29, 30, 38, 41, 42, 43, 44, 46, 50, 51, 52

education and, 38

home settings, 14, 29

levels of care (NICU) and, 13–15

See also Health teaching and health promotion; Neonatal intensive care unit

Workplace issues. *See* Work and practice environments